FAST FACTS

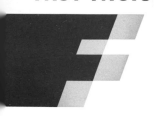

Respiratory Tract Infection

Indispensable

Guides to

Clinical

Practice

Robert C Read
Honorary Consultant Physician
and Senior Lecturer in Infectious Diseases,
Royal Hallamshire Hospital,
Sheffield, UK

James E Pennington
Clinical Professor of Medicine,
Department of Medicine,
University of California,
San Francisco, California,
USA

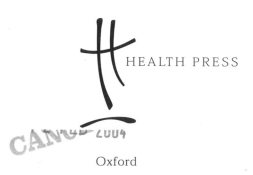

HEALTH PRESS

Oxford

Fast Facts – Respiratory Tract Infection
First published 1998

© 1998 Health Press Limited
Elizabeth House, Queen Street, Abingdon, Oxford OX14 3JR, UK
Tel: +44 (0)1235 523233
Fax: +44 (0)1235 523238

Fast Facts is a trademark of Health Press Limited.

Although every effort has been made to ensure that the drug doses and
other information are presented accurately in this book, the ultimate
responsibility lies with the prescribing physician. The publisher and the
authors cannot accept responsibility for any errors or omissions. Any
product mentioned in this publication should be used in accordance
with the prescribing information supplied by the manufacturers.

A CIP catalogue record for this title is available from the British Library.

ISBN 1-899541-52-7

Library of Congress
Cataloging-in-Publication Data

Read, RC. (Robert)
Fast Facts – Respiratory Tract Infection/
Robert C Read, James E Pennington

Illustrated by Jane Fallows, London, UK

Printed by Fine Print, Oxford, UK

Introduction

Few clinical conditions are as common and as anxiety provoking as respiratory infections. Over 200 million cases of respiratory infection occur annually in the USA alone. While it accounts for only 1–2% of these cases, development of pneumonia is a particular concern to patient and physician alike. Furthermore, the physician is often aware of newly described respiratory pathogens, or emerging antibiotic resistance among previously known pathogens. Add to this the difficulty in reaching a rapid, or in some cases any, specific aetiological diagnosis to guide treatment, and the high morbidity and mortality associated with improper selection of therapy, and the justification for preparing this book is clear. The format is organized to provide quick reference and practical guidelines for busy physicians. However, the use of this manual for practical review by all students of medicine will undoubtedly occur as well. Above all, it is the authors' wish that this publication enhances the quality of clinical care for the patient with respiratory infection.

CHAPTER 1
Community-acquired pneumonia

Pneumonia is a general term used to describe disease that leads to consolidation of the lung parenchyma. It is characterized by acute inflammation within the gas-exchanging areas of the lung with an intense infiltrate of neutrophils in and around the alveoli, and the respiratory and terminal bronchioles. The affected bronchopulmonary segment or entire lobe is consolidated by the resulting inflammation and oedema.

Epidemiology
In the UK, the rate of hospital admissions for pneumonia is approximately 1/1000/year. In the USA, the prevalence is estimated to be 12/1000/year (i.e. approximately 3.3 million cases/year), and bacterial pneumonias account for 500 000 hospital admissions/year of patients aged 15 years or older.

Pneumonia is substantially more common in the winter and affects males more often than females (ratio 2−3:1). It most commonly affects the elderly: in the USA, the incidence of pneumonia requiring hospitalization in those over 75 years of age is 11.6/1000/year compared with 0.54/1000/year in those aged 35−44 years.

Mortality and morbidity
Mortality due to community-acquired pneumonia has decreased markedly since the introduction of antibiotics; the outcome for patients admitted to hospital with pneumonia can be greatly improved by prompt antibiotic therapy. In a study by the British Thoracic Society, none of the patients who died of pneumococcal, staphylococcal or *Mycoplasma pneumoniae* pneumonia had received appropriate antibiotics before hospital admission.

Mortality from ambulatory pneumonia is now about 1% (ambulatory pneumonia is that affecting out-patients/people in the community). In hospitalized patients, however, mortality is approximately 13–15% and, in patients requiring intensive care, it ranges from 22 to 54%.

Patients who survive pneumonia generally recover completely, though there are occasionally long-term sequelae as a result of the development of sepsis syndrome, usually in association with *Streptococcus pneumoniae*, *Legionella pneumophila* or *Klebsiella pneumoniae* infections.

Pathogenesis

Most infections result from initial colonization of the upper respiratory tract by a pathogen, with subsequent translocation by aspiration into the lower airways. The most common cause of community-acquired pneumonia is *S. pneumoniae*, but a wide range of other pathogens may also be implicated (Table 1.1).

Clinical features

In most patients, pneumonia usually develops over several days with cough and sputum production, dyspnoea, pleuritic chest pain, weakness, malaise and often myalgia. Occasionally, the presentation may be hyperacute with a dramatic rigor as the first symptom; this is more common in healthy young

TABLE 1.1

Causes of community-acquired pneumonia*

Pathogen	Cases (%)
Streptococcus pneumoniae	30–54
Haemophilus influenzae	6–15
Influenza A virus	6–9
Mycoplasma pneumoniae	0–18
Legionella pneumophila	2–7
Chlamydia pneumoniae	0–6
Chlamydia psittaci	0–3
Staphylococcus aureus	0–2
Klebsiella pneumoniae	0–2
Streptococcus spp.	0–1
Coxiella burnetii	0–1
Enterobacteriaceae	0–1
Respiratory syncytial virus	0–1

*Data from Meyer RD, Finch RG. *J Hosp Infect* 1992;22(Suppl A):51–9

adults. In older patients, the presentation may be more insidious with minimal cough and absence of fever; confusion and hypothermia are often presenting features in this group.

Physical examination usually reveals fever, particularly in young individuals. Patients are usually uncomfortable and may often be breathless at rest. The trachea is usually central, but expansion on the affected side is reduced. Percussion is dull over the diseased lobe or lobes, and auscultation may reveal rales or bronchial breathing depending on the degree of consolidation. Occasionally, there is evidence of an effusion with stony dullness on the affected side. Typical appearances seen on chest radiography are shown in Figures 1.1–1.4.

In pneumococcal pneumonia, the sputum is classically rusty coloured, but can be mucoid, scanty or absent. In *Mycoplasma* and *Legionella* infections, sputum is usually absent; extrapulmonary symptoms occasionally predominate and can be seen in all patients. Such symptoms include severe headache, confusion, myalgia or polyarthralgia. Until recently, infections in which extrapulmonary symptoms were predominant were considered to be 'atypical pneumonia' and indicative of *Mycoplasma*, *Coxiella* or *Legionella* infection. Now, however, it is accepted that atypical presentations may be seen with pneumococcal pneumonia and the distinction is regarded as unhelpful.

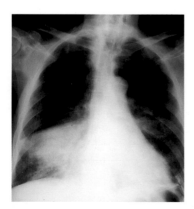

Figure 1.1 Right lower lobe consolidation in a 25-year-old male. *Streptococcus pneumoniae* was isolated in blood cultures.

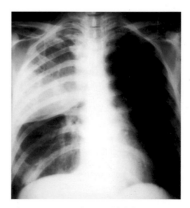

Figure 1.2 Right upper lobe consolidation in a 42-year-old male with *Klebsiella pneumoniae* pneumonia. Note the bulging horizontal fissure.

Figure 1.3 Left lower lobe collapse in an elderly male with left lower lobe pneumonia. Note the retrocardiac shadow and the loss of definition of the left costophrenic angle.

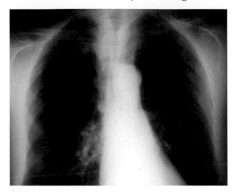

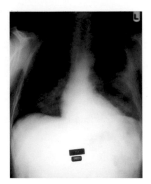

Figure 1.4 Pneumonia due to *Staphylococcus aureus* in an intravenous drug user. Note the evidence of disease in the right lower lobe and abscess formation in the left lower lobe.

Characteristic epidemiological and clinical features, and laboratory abnormalities that may point to a specific microbiological diagnosis are listed in Table 1.2.

Investigations

Investigations that may be indicated include:

- routine haematology and biochemistry
- chest radiograph
- sputum examination and culture (if sputum is expectorated; Figure 1.5)
- alternative methods of obtaining respiratory secretions (e.g. transtracheal aspiration, induced sputum, bronchoalveolar lavage)

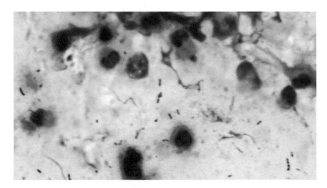

Figure 1.5 Gram stain of sputum from a patient with pneumococcal pneumonia showing pus cells and lancelate Gram-positive cocci.

- blood culture
- acute and convalescent serology to detect antibodies to viruses (including hantaviruses in some localities), *Mycoplasma*, *Chlamydia*, *Legionella* and *Coxiella burnetii*
- urine antigen detection to detect *Legionella* antigen
- aspiration of pleural fluid (for biochemistry and culture)
- cold agglutinins to detect *M. pneumoniae*
- pulse oximetry or blood gases.

Prognosis

A number of clinical and laboratory features are associated with increased mortality in community-acquired pneumonia (Table 1.3). There is a 21-fold increase in the risk of death or the need for admission to an intensive care unit if two or three of the following markers are present:

- respiratory rate above 30 breaths/minute
- diastolic blood pressure below 60 mmHg
- plasma urea level above 7 mmol/litre.

Treatment

Apart from antimicrobial therapy, management of community-acquired pneumonia includes adequate hydration (oral or intravenous), maintenance of arterial blood gases with oxygen therapy or assisted ventilation with continuous positive airway pressure (CPAP) or, if necessary, ventilation.

The British and American Thoracic Societies, as well as the Infectious Diseases Society of America (IDSA), have issued guidelines for the management of adult community-acquired pneumonia (see below). However, if *L. pneumophila* infection is suspected, the patient should be treated with an intravenous macrolide in combination with rifampicin with or without an intravenous fluoroquinolone. If infection with *Staphylococcus aureus* is suspected, the recommended treatment comprises flucloxacillin or nafcillin in combination with fusidic acid.

The British Thoracic Society guidelines for the management of community-acquired pneumonia recommend:

- an aminopenicillin (e.g. oral amoxycillin or intravenous ampicillin) or benzylpenicillin for patients with uncomplicated pneumonia of unknown

11

TABLE 1.2

Characteristic clinical features of pathogens causing community-acquired pneumonia

Pathogen	Epidemiological features	Characteristic clinical features	Characteristic laboratory findings
Streptococcus pneumoniae	Most common cause of community-acquired pneumonia	Unilobar disease, rigors, toxaemia	Gram-positive lancelate cocci in sputum, neutrophil leukocytosis
Mycoplasma pneumoniae	Occurs in 4-yearly cycles	Insidious onset, headache, malaise, myalgia, pharyngitis, otalgia, cough due to peribronchitis, multilobar involvement	Cold agglutinins, convalescent antibody rise
Influenza A virus	Annual winter epidemic	High fever, pharyngitis, bi-basal pneumonia	Convalescent antibody rise, positive PCR or culture of NPA or throat swab
Legionella pneumophila	History of exposure to *Legionella*-contaminated aerosols (e.g. hotel air-conditioning, respiratory therapy equipment)	Gradual onset, malaise, lethargy, fever, headache, myalgia, dry non-productive cough, confusion, hallucinations	Hyponatraemia, abnormal liver function tests, positive urinary antigen, convalescent antibody rise
Coxiella burnetii	History of contact with farm animals	High fever, malaise, headache, dry cough, pleuritic chest pain, prolonged fever	Phase 2 antibody rise

Pathogen	Epidemiological features	Characteristic clinical features	Characteristic laboratory findings
Staphylococcus aureus	Recent influenza infection	Intravenous drug abuse, aggressive and cavitating pneumonia with pleural effusions	Gram-positive cocci in sputum, neutrophil leukocytosis
Klebsiella pneumoniae	Affects alcoholics and the elderly in nursing homes	Aggressive pneumonia, bulging fissure on chest radiograph	Gram-negative bacilli in sputum
Haemophilus influenzae	Affects children and the elderly, especially those in nursing homes	Symptoms preceded by coryza with sudden onset of pleuritic chest pain	
Chlamydia psittaci	Contact with infected birds	Predominant headache and pleuritic pain, dry cough	Convalescent antibody rise
Chlamydia pneumoniae	Affects children in educational institutions and the elderly in nursing homes	Prolonged mild upper and lower respiratory tract symptoms	Convalescent antibody rise
Hantavirus	South-western USA, affects campers, those in contact with rodent faeces	Aggressive pneumonia and sepsis syndrome, with haemoptysis	Detection of antibodies

PCR = polymerase chain reaction; NPA = nasopharyngeal aspirate

TABLE 1.3

Clinical and laboratory features of community-acquired pneumonia associated with increased risk of death*

Clinical features

- Respiratory rate > 30 breaths/minute

- Diastolic blood pressure < 60 mmHg

- Age > 60 years

- Underlying disease

- Confusion

- Atrial fibrillation

- Multilobar involvement

Laboratory features

- Plasma urea > 7 mmol/litre

- Serum albumin < 35 g/litre

- Hypoxaemia with PaO_2 < 8 kPa

- Leukopenia with a WBC < 4 x 10^9/litre

- Leukocytosis with a WBC > 20 x 10^9/litre

- Bacteraemia

WBC = white blood cell count

*Data from Farr BM et al. Ann Intern Med 1991;115:428–36, and Karalus NC et al. Thorax 1991;46:413–18

aetiology without features that indicate severe or non-pneumococcal disease

- the addition of erythromycin to an aminopenicillin in patients with 'atypical' features

- intravenous erythromycin plus a second- or third-generation cephalosporin in severe pneumonia

- erythromycin, or a second- or third-generation cephalosporin in penicillin-allergic patients.

The American Thoracic Society guidelines for the management of community-acquired pneumonia recommend:

- a macrolide or tetracycline in out-patients with no co-morbidity and who are less than 60 years of age

- a second-generation cephalosporin, trimethoprim plus sulphamethoxazole or a beta-lactam with a beta-lactamase inhibitor in out-patients with co-morbidity or who are elderly (i.e. over 60)
- an intravenous second- or third-generation cephalosporin, or a beta-lactam with a beta-lactamase inhibitor for hospitalized patients with community-acquired pneumonia
- an intravenous macrolide plus a third-generation cephalosporin with anti-*Pseudomonas* activity or other anti-*Pseudomonas* agents, such as imipenem or ciprofloxacin, for hospitalized patients with severe community-acquired pneumonia.

The IDSA has published its own guidelines for the management of community-acquired pneumonia (Table 1.4). These are based on more recent data relating to bacterial resistance, and include more modern agents.

Inevitably, each of these guidelines, to some extent, represents opinion rather than fact as there is a dearth of evidence on which the management of community-acquired pneumonia can be based.

Penicillin resistance. *S. pneumoniae* has become more resistant to penicillin over recent years. Strains with intermediate resistance are now prevalent throughout the world and highly resistant isolates are common in certain geographical areas. An oxacillin sensitivity disc is routinely used to screen for penicillin-resistant pneumococci when they are isolated. Such strains are often resistant to other antibiotics, such as chloramphenicol, erythromycin, trimethoprim and clindamycin. In practice, pneumococcal pneumonia almost always responds to penicillin or cephalosporins clinically. Organisms that are highly resistant to high-dose penicillin are susceptible to vancomycin. In future, therapy may require the use of newer agents, including the newer quinolones.

Complications of community-acquired pneumonia

In all patients with community-acquired pneumonia, there is always danger of severe manifestations of sepsis syndrome, including septic shock. Clinical and laboratory features that may suggest such developments include:

- hypotension, particularly refractory hypotension (systolic blood pressure < 100 mmHg, diastolic blood pressure < 60 mmHg)
- oliguria, raised serum creatinine or reduced glomerular filtration rate
- coagulopathy.

15

TABLE 1.4

The Infectious Diseases Society of America's guidelines for the treatment of community-acquired pneumonia

Out-patients

Generally preferred: macrolides*, quinolones[†] or doxycycline

Modifying factors:

- suspected penicillin resistance
  - quinolones[†]
- suspected aspiration
  - co-amoxiclav
- young adult (17–40 years)
  - doxycycline

Hospital in-patients

General medical ward

Generally preferred: beta-lactam[‡] ± macrolides* **or** quinolone[†] (alone)

Alternatives: cefuroxime ± macrolides* **or** azithromycin (alone)

ICU patients with serious pneumonia

Generally preferred: erythromycin, azithromycin **or** a quinolone[†] PLUS cefotaxime, ceftriaxone or beta-lactam/beta-lactamase inhibitor[§]

Modifying factors:

- structural disease of the lung
  - anti-*Pseudomonas* penicillin, a carbapenem **or** cefepime PLUS a macrolide* **or** a quinolone[†] PLUS an aminoglycoside
- penicillin allergy
  - quinolone[†] ± clindamycin
- suspected aspiration
  - quinolone[†] PLUS clindamycin **or** metronidazole
  - quinolone[†] PLUS beta-lactam/beta-lactamase inhibitor

---

* Azithromycin, clarithromycin or erythromycin
† Quinolones with activity against *S. pneumoniae*
‡ Cefotaxime, ceftriaxone or a beta-lactam/beta-lactamase inhibitor
§ Ampicillin/sulbactam or ticaracillin/clavulanate or piperacillin/tazobactam
  (for structural disease of the lung, ticarcillin/clavulanate or piperacillin)

From Bartlett JG *et al*. Community acquired pneumonia in adults: guidelines for management. *Clin Infec Dis* 1998;26:811–38

Patients displaying features such as these should be moved to a high dependency unit and reviewed by intensive care unit physicians.

Empyema is the most common local complication of pneumococcal pneumonia. A reactive effusion can occur but is trivial; empyema is potentially more serious and is presumably due to bacteria reaching the pleural space via the lymphatics. Clinically, this is signalled by the persistence of fever and leukocytosis after 4–5 days of appropriate antibiotic therapy. Empyema is also suggested by large amounts of pleural fluid evident on the chest radiograph. Ultrasound is often useful in determining the site of effusion and identifying the loculae that are typical of empyema (Figure 1.6). Empyema should be drained by repeated needle aspiration or a chest tube; thoracotomy is rarely necessary. Fibrolytic agents, such as urokinase or streptokinase, are being increasingly used to break down loculae.

Lung abscess (see Figure 1.4, page 10) may be detected radiographically as a fluid level within an area of consolidation on the chest radiograph. This can occur in disease due to *S. pneumoniae* and is classically seen in patients with staphylococcal or *Klebsiella* pneumonia. It can occur in patients with a mixed anaerobic infection, for example, as a result of severe dental infection or in patients with pneumonia secondary to aspiration of vomit, such as vagrants with alcoholism or individuals after epileptic fits or cerebrovascular accidents. Management includes surgical drainage and long-term therapy with beta-lactam agents plus an aminoglycoside, or clindamycin plus ciprofloxacin.

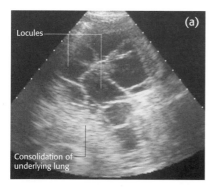
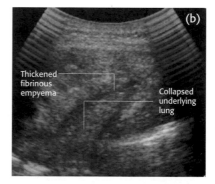

Figure 1.6 Ultrasound images of patients with empyema: (a) note the loculated empyema and the underlying consolidation within lung parenchyma; (b) this patient has thickened, fibrous empyema and a collapsed underlying lung.

Prevention

Case-control field studies have revealed that the 23-valent pneumococcal vaccine has a 56% efficacy in preventing bacteraemic pneumococcal infection. The 23-valent pneumococcal vaccine contains antigens from 23 serotypes of pneumococci that cause most cases of bacteraemic pneumococcal disease; these are serotypes 1, 2, 3, 4, 5, 6B, 7F, 8, 9N, 9V, 10A, 11A, 12F, 14, 15B, 17F, 18C, 19A, 19F, 20, 22F, 23F and 33F. Attempts are underway to increase the clinical efficacy of capsular polysaccharide vaccines by reducing the number of serotypes included in the vaccine (e.g. 9-valent vaccine), and also by the production of conjugated vaccines.

CHAPTER 2

Hospital-acquired pneumonia

Nosocomial pneumonia causes considerable mortality and morbidity, and increases the length of hospital stay and its cost. After urinary tract infection, it is the second most common nosocomial infection.

Definition

The US Centers for Disease Control have defined nosocomial pneumonia as the onset of pneumonia more than 72 hours after hospital admission. It is characterized by lung consolidation or an infiltrate visible on the chest radiograph plus at least one of the following:

- infected sputum
- isolation of a pathogen from the blood, transtracheal aspirate, biopsy or bronchial lavage specimen
- isolation of a virus in respiratory secretions
- diagnostic antibody titres
- histopathological evidence of pneumonia.

Epidemiology

The US National Nosocomial Infections Surveillance System (NISS) identified 0.6–1.0 episodes of nosocomial pneumonia for every 100 hospitalizations occurring in the USA. Nosocomial pneumonia has been shown to affect 18% of postoperative patients. The highest rates of nosocomial pneumonia occur in respiratory and post-surgical ICUs. Infection rates are twice as high in large teaching hospitals compared with smaller institutions, reflecting the association between these infections and high intensity, invasive and interventionist care. The most important factors associated with nosocomial pneumonia are:

- old age
- chronic lung disease
- depressed consciousness
- intubation
- mechanical ventilation
- use of H_2-receptor antagonists

- frequent changes of ventilator circuits
- winter season.

Mortality

Mortality in patients with nosocomial pneumonia is high (20–50%), though only about one-third of the deaths are directly due to the pneumonia. Again, this reflects the fact that these infections occur primarily in the most sick and vulnerable hospitalized patients.

Pathogenesis

The first step in the pathogenesis of nosocomial pneumonia is colonization of the upper airways of hospitalized patients by potential pathogens. The probable routes of this contamination are summarized in Figure 2.1. Patients admitted to ICUs become colonized by aerobic Gram-negative bacilli within 1 week of entering hospital and, of these, about 25% develop nosocomial pneumonia. There is a direct correlation between severity of illness in hospitalized patients and the likelihood of development of nosocomial pneumonia. Enterobacteriaceae probably reach the upper respiratory tract by faecal–oral transmission. On the other hand, *Pseudomonas aeruginosa* and *S. aureus* probably colonize patients from environmental sources through contamination of respiratory devices or other supporting equipment by attending staff.

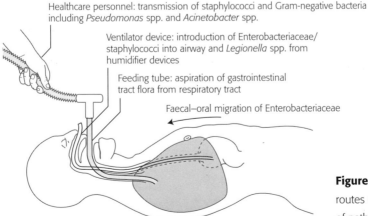

Healthcare personnel: transmission of staphylococci and Gram-negative bacteria including *Pseudomonas* spp. and *Acinetobacter* spp.

Ventilator device: introduction of Enterobacteriaceae/staphylococci into airway and *Legionella* spp. from humidifier devices

Feeding tube: aspiration of gastrointestinal tract flora from respiratory tract

Faecal–oral migration of Enterobacteriaceae

Figure 2.1 Probable routes of transmission of pathogens leading to nosocomial pneumonia.

Microbial aetiology

Polymicrobial infections are common. Most nosocomial pneumonias are caused by aerobic Gram-negative bacilli or staphylococci (Table 2.1). Other less common causes of nosocomial pneumonia include:

- fungi (including *Candida*)
- viruses
- *Acinetobacter* (especially in the intensive care setting)
- *L. pneumophila* (especially during hospital outbreaks)
- *Mycobacterium tuberculosis*
- anaerobic bacteria (especially in severe aspiration).

The precise microbial aetiology of nosocomial pneumonia differs from institution to institution, and the microbiological yield also varies according to the diagnostic methodology used. The microbial aetiology of the pneumonia also leads to differences in the mortality rate (Table 2.2).

TABLE 2.1

Most common causes of nosocomial pneumonia

Pathogen	Prevalence (%)
Enterobacteriaceae (*Enterobacter* spp., *Klebsiella* spp., *Escherichia coli, Serratia marcescens*)	40
Staphylococcus aureus	25
Pseudomonas aeruginosa	15
Haemophilus influenzae	6

TABLE 2.2

Variation in the mortality of nosocomial pneumonia due to different infecting pathogens

Microbial aetiology	Reported mortality (%)
Aerobic Gram-negative organisms	50
Gram-positive organisms	5–25
Pseudomonas aeruginosa	70–80
Legionella pneumophila	50

A number of risk factors can predispose patients to infection with particular pathogens, and this can assist the clinical evaluation of an individual patient and influence the choice of empirical antimicrobial therapy (Table 2.3).

TABLE 2.3

Risk factors predisposing to different microbial aetiologies in nosocomial pneumonia

Staphylococcus aureus

- Diabetes
- Elderly
- Renal failure
- Recent influenza
- Recent head injury
- Trauma

Pseudomonas aeruginosa

- Malnourishment
- Steroid treatment
- Chronic lung disease
- Prolonged mechanical ventilation
- Prolonged intensive care

Legionella pneumophila

- Immunosuppression
- Steroid treatment
- Contamination of hospital water facilities

Anaerobes

- Recent thoraco-abdominal surgery
- Gross aspiration

Viruses (RSV, influenza A, para-influenza, adenovirus)

- Young age (0–5 years)

Haemophilus influenzae

- Chronic lung disease

Diagnosis

Outside the ICU, a clinical diagnosis can be made relatively easily based on fever, cough and sputum production together with the appearance of new infiltrates on the chest radiograph. In patients receiving intensive care, however, the diagnosis of nosocomial pneumonia can be difficult and is often confused with adult respiratory distress syndrome (ARDS). In addition, isolation of potential pathogens (e.g. *Candida* spp.) from respiratory tract aspirate may imply colonization rather than disease. Clinical parameters that may indicate the onset of nosocomial pneumonia in such patients include:

- an increase in the quantity and purulence of respiratory secretions
- a rapid change in infiltrates seen on chest radiography
- a reduction in $Pa\mathrm{O}_2$
- a rapid increase in amount of oxygen required to maintain arterial oxygen level
- a change in fever pattern
- the absence of other events that might explain these changes (e.g. ARDS, haemorrhage, pulmonary embolism, lung contusion, atelectasis).

Investigations employed in the diagnosis of nosocomial pneumonia in severely ill patients may include transtracheal aspiration, bronchoscopic sampling with or without protected brush, and transcutaneous aspiration of lung material. In many studies, however, these techniques have not been shown to be superior to traditional clinical and radiological evaluation, in terms of risk and cost benefit.

In patients outside the ICU, sputum production may yield Gram-positive (*S. aureus*) or Gram-negative bacteria. In intubated patients, aspirated respiratory secretions and blood cultures (bacteraemia occurs in approximately 2–6% of nosocomial pneumonias) may provide a bacteriological diagnosis without the need for invasive investigation. In most cases, however, decisions regarding antimicrobial therapy need to be taken without a precise microbiological diagnosis.

Treatment

If the pathogen is known, antimicrobial therapy should be guided by the antibiotic sensitivities. Empirical therapy should include antibiotics active against *S. aureus* and Gram-negative bacteria. However, therapy may need to be modified in certain situations, for example when:

- *P. aeruginosa* is likely (e.g. in mechanically ventilated patients or those receiving steroids)
- *Haemophilus influenzae* is suspected (e.g. in patients with chronic lung disease)
- *L. pneumophila* infection is a possibility (e.g. during hospital outbreaks).

Empirical regimens commonly used to treat nosocomial pneumonia are listed in Table 2.4. In patients in ICUs and those who develop nosocomial pneumonia following instigation of mechanical ventilation, however, it is necessary to use empirical therapy that takes into account the likelihood of infection with *P. aeruginosa* and other highly resistant organisms including *Serratia marcescens* and *Acinetobacter*. Common regimens include:

- ceftazidime plus an aminoglycoside
- ceftazidime plus clindamycin
- ciprofloxacin plus clindamycin
- a broad-spectrum penicillin plus an aminoglycoside.

Monotherapies. Although empirical monotherapy has been reported to have equivalent efficacy to combination therapy in severe nosocomial pneumonia, there is danger of resistance developing during therapy, especially with infections due to *P. aeruginosa*. Suitable monotherapies include:

- a broad-spectrum penicillin plus beta-lactamase inhibitor (e.g. ticarcillin plus clavulanic acid or piperacillin/tazobactam)
- cephalosporin with anti-*Pseudomas* activity (e.g. ceftazidime or cefepime)
- imipenem or meropenem
- ciprofloxacin.

If respiratory secretions or blood culture yield positive microbiology, antibiotic therapy can be modified to take account of the sensitivities of the organism identified. However, in view of the polymicrobial nature of this disease, it is traditional in practice to continue with broad-spectrum cover.

Prevention

Prevention of nosocomial pneumonia depends on limiting colonization and aspiration, and the spread of pathogens between patients and staff.

Measures that have been shown to be effective include:

- handwashing by hospital staff
- restriction of oral intake of fluid and nutrients if swallowing is impaired
- avoiding unnecessary nasogastric or endotracheal intubation

---

TABLE 2.4

Empirical regimens used in the treatment of nosocomial pneumonia

Moderately ill patients able to take oral medication

- Oral co-amoxiclav
- Aminopenicillin plus flucloxacillin or nafcillin
- Ciprofloxacin or ofloxacin
- Oral ciprofloxacin or ofloxacin, plus clindamycin

Severely ill patients (intravenous therapy)

All patients

- Nafcillin (flucloxacillin) plus aminoglycoside
- Second-generation cephalosporin plus aminoglycoside
- Clindamycin plus aminoglycoside
- Broad-spectrum penicillin plus aminoglycoside
- Broad-spectrum penicillin plus beta-lactamase inhibitor
- Quinolone

Patients with chronic lung disease (Haemophilus influenzae a likely co-pathogen)

- Second- or third-generation cephalosporin plus aminoglycoside
- Quinolone

Following aspiration (anaerobes)

- Aminopenicillin plus metronidazole plus aminoglycoside
- Clindamycin plus quinolone
- Third-generation cephalosporin plus aminoglycoside
- Clindamycin plus ciprofloxacin

Patients in hospitals where Legionella pneumophila is endemic

- Macrolide plus quinolone
- Macrolide plus rifampicin plus quinolone

- elevation of the patient's head to reduce risk of aspiration
- avoiding the use of H_2-receptor antagonists in seriously ill patients
- substitution of sucralfate for H_2-receptor antagonists to prevent erosive gastritis.

A number of other measures to prevent nosocomial pneumonia have been evaluated, but have had limited efficacy. Such measures include the use of prophylactic endobronchial antibiotics, selective decontamination of the digestive tract with broad-spectrum antibiotics and antifungal agents, and immunoprophylaxis with lipopolysaccharide (LPS) vaccine.

CHAPTER 3

Infective exacerbation of chronic obstructive pulmonary disease

Chronic obstructive pulmonary disease (COPD) is characterized by airflow obstruction due to chronic bronchitis or emphysema; this is defined as a ratio of forced expiratory volume in 1 second:forced vital capacity (FEV_1:FVC) of less than 70%. The decline in FEV_1 with advancing age is much greater in patients with COPD than in normal individuals, and is particularly rapid in those patients who continue to smoke (Figure 3.1). Infective exacerbations are also associated with an acute decline in FEV_1. Although infection is the most common cause of death in patients with COPD, it is unclear whether infectious exacerbations lead to an accelerated loss of lung function during the natural history of chronic bronchitis.

Epidemiology

In contrast to heart disease and cerebrovascular disease, the incidence and prevalence of COPD are increasing. In the USA, COPD is the fourth leading cause of death, affecting 14% of adult men and 8% of adult women; UK figures are similar. Infective exacerbations of COPD are common during the winter months and occur, on average, three times per year.

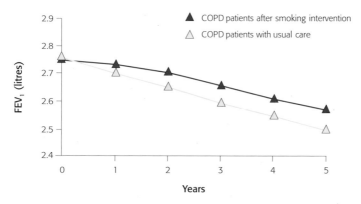

Figure 3.1 The accelerated decline in FEV_1 in individuals with COPD is greatest in individuals who continue to smoke. Data from Anthonisen NR, Connett JE, Kiley JP *et al.* JAMA 1994; 272:1497–505.

COPD has a significant economic impact. In the UK, chronic bronchitis is associated with a loss of 28 million working days/year. In addition to this, COPD accounts for a large proportion of the £42 million ($75 million) spent on antibiotic prescriptions for lower respiratory tract infections every year in the UK.

Pathology

The underlying pathology of stable COPD is airway remodelling as a consequence of chronic airways narrowing. In emphysema, the chronic airflow limitation is due to destruction of the alveolar structures, while in chronic bronchitis, it is due to chronic inflammation secondary to mucous gland hypertrophy and hyperplasia, and peribronchial fibrosis.

In infective exacerbations of COPD, purulent sputum most commonly yields:

- *H. influenzae*
- *S. pneumoniae*
- *Moraxella catarrhalis.*

Indeed, these organisms are present in many patients between exacerbations and their number simply increases during the infective episode. In most cases, the initiating factor of an infective exacerbation is unknown, but viral and *Mycoplasma* infections are responsible for up to one-third of the acute exacerbations of COPD; the viruses most commonly identified include influenza A, para-influenza virus, coronavirus and rhinovirus.

H. influenzae has tropism for airway epithelium and attaches to the airway mucosa that is damaged in patients with COPD (Figure 3.2). It adheres to mucus via pili, and to galactoside sequences on the epithelial cells. Soluble products of *H. influenzae* have been shown to reduce ciliary

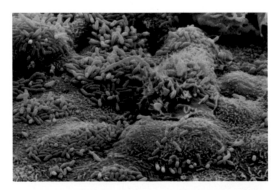

Figure 3.2 Scanning electron microscopy of human airway mucosa showing adherence of *Haemophilus influenzae* to the surface epithelial cells (RC Read and A Brain).

beat frequency and mucociliary clearance. In patients with more severe disease, Gram-negative bacilli (including *P. aeruginosa*) and *S. aureus* can be recovered from purulent sputum.

Clinical features

Patients with COPD usually present as a result of an infective exacerbation of the disease, and usually have one or more of the following symptoms:

- increased dyspnoea
- increased sputum volume
- increased sputum purulence.

Between exacerbations, patients have exercise limitation as a result of their airways obstruction. This can be staged according to the FEV_1 (Table 3.1).

Investigations

The diagnosis is usually clinically obvious, but investigations necessary in severely ill patients include:

- chest radiograph
- biochemical tests
- haematology
- formal blood gas analysis
- measurement of peak expiratory flow (PEF) and formal spirometry
- sputum culture
- blood culture.

Culture of sputum is of doubtful value in some patients, because it is likely to be contaminated by pathogens that are also present in oropharyngeal secretions. It is therefore important to ensure that only purulent sputum is obtained.

TABLE 3.1

Staging of chronic obstructive pulmonary disease

FEV_1 (% predicted value)	Degree	Stage
> 50	Moderate	I
35–49	Severe	II
< 35	Very severe	III

Prognostic indicators

Factors associated with increased morbidity and mortality include:

- decreased lung function (FEV_1 < 1.0 litre)
- blood gas changes – worsening hypercapnia (especially when cardiac disease is present)
- co-morbid conditions
- frequent exacerbations
- mucus hypersecretion
- continued smoking
- malnutrition
- treatment with corticosteroids
- increasing age (> 70 years).

Management of COPD

The general management of patients with COPD between infective exacerbations includes:

- encouragement to stop smoking
- respiratory rehabilitation (physiological training: graded physical exercises and breathing exercises)
- long-term oxygen therapy
- drug treatment.

Drug treatment. A step-wise pharmacological management programme of COPD has been suggested by Celli.

- Intermittent symptoms should be treated with beta-agonists as required.
- Mild persistent symptoms should be treated with ipratropium plus beta-agonists as required.
- Severe persistent symptoms should be treated with a combination of ipratropium, beta-agonists and theophylline as required; theophylline should be monitored.
- A COPD crisis should be treated with ipratropium and beta-agonists as required, together with a trial of corticosteroids.

Antibiotic therapy. The effect of antibiotics on the outcome of exacerbations in COPD has been assessed in a number of trials. In general, these have shown a small benefit in this heterogenous population (Table 3.2).

TABLE 3.2

Results of trials to assess the effect of antibiotics on the outcome of exacerbations in chronic obstructive pulmonary disease

Source	Setting	Total number of patients	Treatment	Main outcome measure	Effect on outcome
Elmes et al. 1957	Out-patient	130	Oxytetracycline	Days of illness	Small reduction compared with placebo
Fear and Edwards 1962	Out-patient	119	Oxytetracycline	Overall score by physician	Moderate improvement compared with placebo
Pines et al. 1972	In-patient	149	Tetracycline	Overall physician score/change in PEF	Moderate improvement compared with placebo
Anthonisen et al. 1987	Out-patient	310	Trimethoprim– sulphamethoxazole, amoxycillin, doxycycline	Days of illness Change in PEF	Moderate benefit in patients with most severe illness only
Jorgensen et al. 1992	Out-patient	262	Amoxycillin	Overall score by physician/ change in PEF	Minimal effect compared with placebo

PEF = peak expiratory flow
Adapted from Saint S et al. JAMA 1995;273:957–60

The systematic review by Saint *et al.* (1995) of 1101 patients with acute exacerbations demonstrated a significant, although small, positive effect of antibiotics compared with placebo in terms of simple clinical evidence of improvement and peak expiratory flow rate.

Anthonisen *et al.* demonstrated that when patients were stratified according to severity of their exacerbations, there was a clear improvement in clinical outcome with antibiotic therapy in those with the most severe illness (those with at least two out of three of increased dyspnoea, sputum volume and sputum purulence). In view of this, Wilson has suggested a simple classification system for the use of antibiotic therapy in COPD that takes into account the baseline clinical status, prognostic markers and likely pathogens (Table 3.3). Simple antibiotic therapy (e.g. an oral aminopenicillin) is recommended for patients with uncomplicated illness,

TABLE 3.3

Empiric classifications of patients with chronic bronchitis and suggested therapy

Baseline clinical status	Presenting clinical features
Acute tracheobronchitis	No underlying structural disease
Simple chronic bronchitis	$FEV_1 > 50\%$ Increased sputum volume and purulence
Complicated chronic bronchitis	$FEV_1 < 50\%$ Advanced age $\geq$ Four exacerbations/year Significant co-morbid disease
Chronic bronchial suppuration (bronchiectasis)	Stage III plus continuous purulent sputum production

FEV_1 = forced expiratory volume in 1 second
Adapted from Wilson R. Chest 1995;108:52S–7S

but patients who are older, with poor underlying lung function (FEV$_1$ $\leq$ 50% predicted) or co-morbid illness, are more likely to have had recurrent courses of antimicrobials and be colonized by resistant organisms. Therefore, in this group, treatment with relatively sophisticated antimicrobials, including amoxycillin–clavulanic acid, ciprofloxacin, second- or third-generation cephalosporins or modern macrolides, is indicated in order to ensure adequate eradication of *H. influenzae*.

Hospitalization is necessary for patients with an acute exacerbation of COPD, characterized by increased dyspnoea, cough and sputum production, who have:
- failed to respond to out-patient management
- acute immobility

Pathogens	Suggested antibiotic therapy
Usually viral	None
Haemophilus influenzae, Moraxella catarrhalis, Streptococcus pneumoniae (possible beta-lactam resistance)	Either none, or simple beta-lactam therapy
Haemophilus influenzae, Moraxella catarrhalis, Streptococcus pneumoniae (resistance to beta-lactams common)	Amoxycillin–clavulanic acid, quinolone, second- or third-generation cephalosporins, modern macrolide
As with complicated chronic bronchitis plus Enterobacteriaceae, *Pseudomonas aeruginosa*	High-dose aminopenicillin, high-dose second- or third-generation cephalosporin, high-dose quinolone

- inability to eat or sleep due to dyspnoea
- high-risk co-morbid conditions (e.g. pneumonia, heart failure, cor pulmonale)
- new or worsening hypercapnia or hypoxaemia.

Patients who are severely ill may require assisted ventilation including nasal CPAP to support gas exchange. Intubation should not be withheld from patients who have not been ventilated before, because their prognosis is relatively good.

CHAPTER 4

Pulmonary tuberculosis

Pulmonary tuberculosis is now re-emerging as a significant problem in developed countries. This is a reversal of the decline in the incidence of the disease, and the consequent reduction in mortality, seen between the 1940s and the 1970s. The positive influence of improvements in social welfare and the development of effective anti-tuberculous agents has been counteracted by problems of AIDS, urban decline and overcrowding, immigration and the spectre of multidrug-resistant *Mycobacterium tuberculosis*.

Epidemiology

Approximately one-third of the world's population of 1.7 billion has been infected by *M. tuberculosis* at some time. Of the 100 million people who become infected every year, about 10% will develop tuberculosis and many will die as a result. In 1994, approximately 3 million people (a third of whom were children) died of tuberculosis. Furthermore, the annual incidence of tuberculosis in most developed countries is rising; figures published by the WHO showed a rise of 5–30% between 1989 and 1992.

The worldwide distribution of cases of tuberculosis is shown in Figure 4.1. The prevalence of HIV is a significant epidemiological factor in areas with a high incidence of tuberculosis. In sub-Saharan Africa, almost 50% of individuals in the age group most susceptible to HIV infection (15–45 years) are infected with *M. tuberculosis*, compared with about 12% in the USA and Western Europe.

Pathogenesis

The *Mycobacterium tuberculosis* complex is dominated by two closely related species – *M. tuberculosis* and *M. bovis*. *M. tuberculosis* is mainly transmitted by droplet spread from patients with cough. *M. bovis* remains a problem in areas where agricultural control measures have not been instituted and is spread to farm workers by diseased cattle or to urban dwellers in unpasteurized milk.

Transmission occurs almost exclusively via patients whose sputum is smear-positive (i.e. contains 5000 bacilli/ml). Approximately 10% of

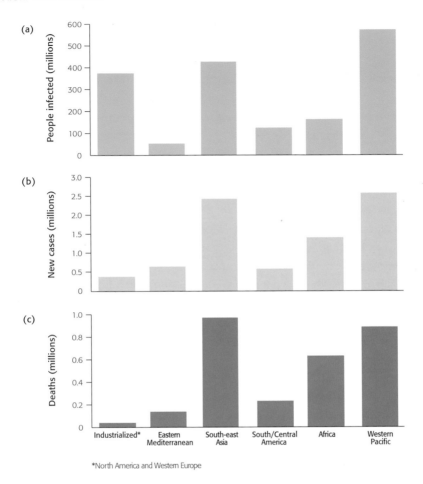

Figure 4.1 Estimated worldwide (a) incidence, (b) prevalence, and (c) mortality of tuberculosis in 1991. Data from Kochi A. The Global Tuberculosis Situation and the New Control Strategy of the WHO. *Tubercle* 1991;72:1–6.

non-immunocompromised individuals who become infected eventually develop overt disease. Of these, 50% will develop 'primary disease' (i.e. within 5 years of infection), while the other 50% will develop 'post-primary disease'. Once inhaled, *M. tuberculosis* is taken up by macrophages, but normal lung macrophages are incapable of killing *M. tuberculosis* and require activation by CD4+ cells via interferon (IFN)-γ. Activated macrophages aggregate to form characteristic granulomas, which together with a lymphocytic infiltrate produce IFN-γ and other cytokines, including tumour necrosis factor (TNF).

Tubercle bacilli are destroyed by a combination of intracellular killing and the anoxia within the middle of the granuloma that results from necrosis.

Approximately 95% of primarily infected individuals kill tubercle bacilli by this mechanism, though some bacilli may survive for years in a dormant state. If bacilli are not effectively killed locally, they are transported to regional lymph nodes and are taken up by dendritic cells for antigen presentation. Other bacilli disseminate throughout the body, including the CNS.

Clinical features

Primary tuberculosis. Primary disease, seldom seen in Western Europe and the USA, consists of an initial febrile illness with erythema nodosum and/or phlyctenular conjunctivitis. Within 12 months of the primary infection, complications of the Ghon focus, including pleural effusion, empyema and bronchopneumonia, may develop. This may be followed by regional lymphadenopathy, including lobar collapse, tuberculous bronchopneumonia and pericardial effusion, which can occur within 2 years of the primary infection, and meningitis and osteomyelitis within 3 years. Late complications, which may appear up to 5 years after the primary infection, include renal and skin disease.

Post-primary tuberculosis ('adult type'). Post-primary disease occurs 5 years or more after the primary infection and develops in only 5% of those infected. It is characterized by extensive tissue necrosis, classically involving the upper lobes of the lung. This is the result of tissue-necrotizing hypersensitivity that is quite distinct from the protective immune reactions seen in most affected individuals. Infected tissue in patients with post-primary tuberculosis is extremely sensitive to necrosis induced by TNF-α and is probably the result of priming by cytokines associated with the type 2 T-helper lymphocyte (Th2) cell maturation pathway.

The main features of post-primary pulmonary tuberculosis are:
- fever and sweating
- cough producing mucoid or purulent sputum
- haemoptysis
- chest wall pain
- dyspnoea
- weight loss, lassitude, anorexia

- apical crackles, apical bronchial breathing or wheeze
- pleural effusion
- clubbing.

The radiological features are shown in Figure 4.2.

Diagnosis

Pulmonary tuberculosis is diagnosed following the identification of the organism in a suitable specimen. Such specimens include:

- sputum (expectorated or induced)
- laryngeal swabs
- gastric aspirates after overnight fasting
- pleural fluid
- bronchoalveolar lavage
- blood.

Methods of detecting *Mycobacteria* include microscopic examination, culture and radiometric techniques.

The simplest of these is microscopic examination following Ziehl-Neelsen staining (Figure 4.3), or fluorescent staining with auramine (Figure 4.4) or rhodamine B. This provides a rapid diagnosis of infection with *Mycobacterium* spp.

Culture methods consist of decontamination of the clinical material (to remove oropharyngeal flora – various disinfectants can be used), followed

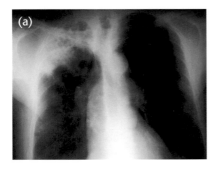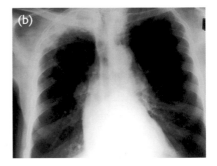

Figure 4.2 (a) Pulmonary tuberculosis in a 47-year-old male immigrant from the Indian subcontinent. In the right upper lobe, there is consolidation with cavitation; (b) after 3 months' therapy with anti-tuberculous chemotherapy. Note residual fibrosis in the right apex.

Figure 4.3 Ziehl-Neelsen stain of sputum from the patient described previously (Figure 4.2). The acid-fast bacilli (in the centre of the field) are stained pink against a blue background.

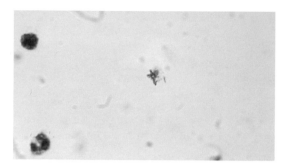

by incubation on Lowenstein's media. Inoculated media are incubated for at least 8 weeks and inspected weekly for growth. Most strains of *Mycobacterium* tuberculosis complex produce visible colonies after 4 – 6 weeks, and are clearly identifiable by their slow growth rate, lack of pigment, temperature sensitivity and sensitivity to *p*-nitrobenzoic acid. Although this technique provides accurate culture diagnosis and sensitivities, it is slow.

Modern radiometric techniques permit detection of *Mycobacteria* within 2 weeks. Clinical material is inoculated into Middlebrook 12B broth containing antibiotics and then labelled with radiolabelled palmitic acid. If *Mycobacteria* are present, $^{14}CO_2$ is liberated and detected radiometrically (Figure 4.5).

DNA amplification by PCR, and amplification techniques for mycobacterial ribosomal RNA are rapidly evolving. These techniques provide quick results, and may even allow rapid prediction of antimicrobial sensitivity.

Serodiagnostic techniques have been disappointing because of lack of specificity.

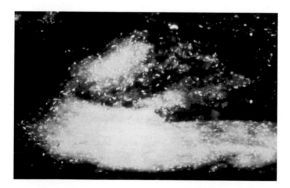

Figure 4.4 Auramine stain of sputum from patient with tuberculosis showing epifluorescence of bacilli. Reproduced courtesy of Dr E Ridgway, Royal Hallamshire Hospital, Sheffield, UK.

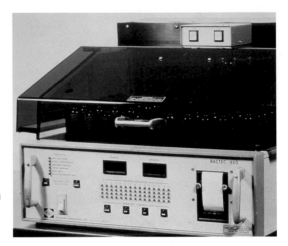

Figure 4.5 Modern methods of culture of *Mycobacterium tuberculosis* employ radiometric techniques that can detect viable *Mycobacteria* more quickly than conventional culture on solid media. Reproduced with permission from Becton-Dickinson.

Tuberculin testing measures an individual's sensitivity to tuberculin protein, and conversion from a negative to a positive tuberculin test indicates recent infection. A number of factors may depress reactivity including:

- advanced disease
- old age
- malnutrition
- immunosuppression including that caused by HIV infection
- intrinsic 'poor reactors'
- infectious mononucleosis and other recent viral infections
- recent administration of live viral vaccines
- sarcoidosis
- corticosteroid therapy.

Mantoux test. In the Mantoux test, 0.1 ml containing 10 IU of purified protein derivative (PPD), or 1 IU PPD in people likely to react strongly, is injected intracutaneously and the diameter of the resulting induration is measured 48–72 hours later. Reactions more than 10 mm in diameter are positive; those between 5 and 9 mm are doubtful positive.

Heaf test. In the Heaf test, a re-usable Heaf gun with a disposable head propels six needles into the skin to a depth of 2 mm through a drop of undiluted PPD (100 000 IU/ml). The test is read after 72 hours and graded accordingly (Figure 4.6). A Heaf reaction of at least grade II is regarded as positive.

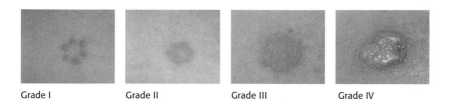

Grade I   Grade II   Grade III   Grade IV

Figure 4.6 Grading of the Heaf test. Grade I – four or more papules at puncture sites; Grade II – confluence of the papules into a ring; Grade III – a single large plaque; Grade IV – a plaque with vesicle formation or central necrosis. Reproduced with permission from Dr JA Lunn.

Treatment

Experience in the 1950s showed that long periods of therapy with multiple drugs are necessary to avoid relapse caused by the development of resistance. The efficacy of standard chemotherapeutic agents against the functionally different tubercle bacilli is shown in Figure 4.7.

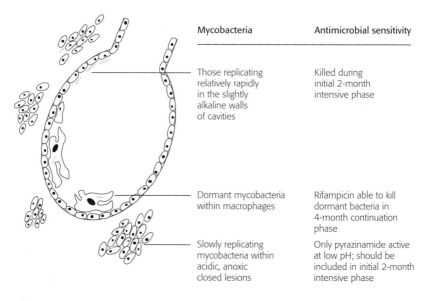

Mycobacteria	Antimicrobial sensitivity
Those replicating relatively rapidly in the slightly alkaline walls of cavities	Killed during initial 2-month intensive phase
Dormant mycobacteria within macrophages	Rifampicin able to kill dormant bacteria in 4-month continuation phase
Slowly replicating mycobacteria within acidic, anoxic closed lesions	Only pyrazinamide active at low pH; should be included in initial 2-month intensive phase

Figure 4.7 Lung infected with *Mycobacterium tuberculosis* contains at least three functionally distinct mycobacteria with differing sensitivities to antimicrobial agents. Adapted from Grange JM. Tuberculosis. In: Collier L, Balows A, Sussman M, eds. *Topley & Wilson's Systematic Bacteriology,* ninth edition. London: Arnold, 1998:391–418.

41

Recommended drug regimens (Table 4.1) consist of an intense 2-month treatment phase in which all but the near-dormant intra-macrophage bacilli are killed. This is followed by a 4-month continuation phase to eradicate the remaining organisms. The standard regimen recommended by WHO is a short course of directly observed therapy (DOTS). While DOTS ensures compliance, it does require frequent contact between the patient and physician.

The doses and side-effects of commonly used drugs are shown in Table 4.2.

Side-effects. Dangerous hepatotoxicity caused by rifampicin, isoniazid or pyrazinamide can be prevented by regular monitoring of liver function, and interruption of therapy if transaminase levels rise above four times normal. Isoniazid neurotoxicity is avoided by administration of pyridoxine (vitamin B_6). Retinopathy associated with ethambutol is possible, but unlikely, at doses of 15 mg/kg or below; it is reversible and can be avoided by regular optometry. Streptomycin (or amikacin) nephrotoxicity and ototoxicity can be avoided by monitoring blood levels and renal function. All patients should be warned about the reduction in efficacy of oral contraceptives during rifampicin therapy (due to induction of cytochrome isoenzymes).

Drug-resistant tuberculosis. Factors that may point to the possibility of infection with an organism that is resistant to first-line agents include:

TABLE 4.1

Drug regimens for tuberculosis recommended by the WHO

	Intensive phase (2 months)	Continuation phase (4 months)
Standard regimen – directly observed therapy, short course (DOTS)	EHRZ daily	HR three times/week
	HRZ daily	HR daily
	SHRZ daily	HR daily
	EHRZ daily	HR daily
Intermittent regimens	SHRZ three times/week	HRZ three times/week
	EHRZ three times/week	HRZ three times/week

E = ethambutol; H = isoniazid; R = rifampicin; Z = pyrazinamide; S = streptomycin

- recent immigration from an area with high incidence of multiple-drug resistant (MDR) tuberculosis (e.g. Pakistan, South-east Asia)
- clinical deterioration despite appropriate therapy
- history of poor compliance.

In the simple case of a patient from a high-risk area with newly diagnosed tuberculosis, the US Advisory Council for the Elimination of Tuberculosis recommends:

- administration of one of the four drug regimens outlined in Table 4.1, under direct supervision
- rapid radiometric techniques to determine whether the isolate is resistant.

If the organism is proved to be resistant, or there is strong clinical evidence of deterioration in a patient receiving therapy with three or four drugs, then at least three second-line agents to which the patient has not been previously exposed should be employed (Table 4.3). Patients with confirmed MDR tuberculosis should continue treatment for 18–24 months.

Prophylactic therapy

Isoniazid monotherapy can be given as prophylaxis on the grounds that it is relatively well tolerated and, in most circumstances, patients will be infected with relatively few bacilli, with consequently less likelihood of resistance developing. Appropriate recipients include:

- individuals who have recently converted to tuberculin test positive
- breast-fed infants with sputum-positive mothers
- tuberculin reactors under 35 years of age (in the USA)
- all tuberculin-positive HIV-infected individuals.

Prophylactic isoniazid is given at a dose of 5 mg/kg/day up to a maximum of 300 mg/day for 6–12 months.

Bacille Calmette-Guérin (BCG) vaccine contains a live, attenuated strain of *M. bovis*. Its efficacy varies remarkably from country to country, but in children in the UK, it has a protective efficacy of 70–80% over at least 15 years; it is not advocated for routine use in the USA.

BCG is administered to:

- in the UK, all individuals who are tuberculin-negative, and have no characteristic BCG scar (a tuberculin test is conducted nationwide at age 12–13 years)

TABLE 4.2

Doses and adverse effects of drugs commonly used to treat tuberculosis

Drug	Daily dose		Intermittent dose
	Adults	Children	Adults
Isoniazid	300 mg (chemoprophylaxis 5 mg/kg)	10 mg/kg	15 mg/kg (max 750 mg) plus pyridoxine, 10 mg
Rifampicin	< 50 kg: 450 mg > 50 kg: 600 mg	10 mg/kg (max 600 mg)	600–900 mg
Pyrazinamide	< 50 kg: 1.5 g 50–75 kg: 2.0 g > 75 kg: 2.5 g	35 mg/kg	*Three times/week* < 50 kg: 2.0 g > 50 kg: 2.5 g *Twice/week* < 50 kg: 3.0 g > 50 kg: 3.5 g
Ethambutol	15 mg/kg	If over 12 years of age, as adults	*Three times/week* 30 mg/kg *Twice/week* 45 mg/kg
Streptomycin	< 50 kg: 0.75 g > 50 kg: 1.0 g or 0.75 g if over 40 years of age	20 mg/kg	< 50 kg: 0.75 g > 50 kg: 1.0 g
Thioacetazone	150 mg	4 mg/kg	Unsuitable

	Common side-effects	Drug interactions
Children		
15 mg/kg (max 750 mg) plus pyridoxine, 10 mg daily	Peripheral neuropathy; cutaneous hypersensitivity; hepatitis; elevation of hepatic enzymes	Phenytoin
10 mg/kg (max 600 mg)	Nausea and vomiting; hepatitis; toxic reactions in intermittent therapy; orange body secretions	Oral contraceptives; coumarin drugs; corticosteroids; digoxin; oral hypoglycaemics; methadone
Three times/week 50 mg/kg *Twice/week* 75 mg/kg	Hepatitis; arthralgia (hyperuricaemia); photosensitivity; nausea; anorexia; vomiting	
If over 12 years of age, as adults	Retinopathy (dose related)	Potentiation of neuromuscular-blocking agents
20 mg/kg (max 0.75 g)	Giddiness; ataxia; tinnitus; ototoxicity; nephrotoxicity; avoid pregnancy	
Unsuitable	Nausea and vomiting; cutaneous reaction (often severe); conjunctivitis	

TABLE 4.3

Treatment of drug-resistant tuberculosis: second-line agents

Agent	Dose	Common adverse events
Ethionamide Prothionamide	< 50 kg: 750 mg in divided doses (to avoid nausea) > 50 kg: 1 g	Gastrointestinal; metallic taste in mouth
Sodium para-aminosalicylate (PAS)	10–12 g/day divided into two equal doses	Gastrointestinal; fever; rash
Cycloserine	250 mg twice/day increasing to 250 mg three times/day	Confusion; convulsions; suicide
Aminoglycosides (kanamycin, viomycin)	< 50 kg: 0.75 g > 50 kg: 1.0 g or 0.75 g if over 40 years of age Monitor serum urea, serum creatinine and electrolyte concentrations	As for streptomycin, but ototoxicity less common
Capreomycin	As for aminoglycosides	
Ciprofloxacin	250–500 mg twice/day	Relatively well tolerated

- health professionals
- vets
- prison staff
- contacts of patients with active tuberculosis who have two consecutive negative tuberculin tests.

BCG is contraindicated in:

- patients receiving corticosteroids or other immunosuppressive therapy
- HIV-infected individuals
- haematological malignancies
- pregnant women.

CHAPTER 5

Bronchiectasis and cystic fibrosis

Bronchiectasis

Bronchiectasis refers to irreversible abnormal dilatation of the bronchi, accompanied by suppurative inflammation that is subject to infective exacerbations. Thickened, infected mucus is produced continuously and this must be expectorated in order to prevent exacerbations developing. During an infective exacerbation, large quantities of purulent sputum are produced. The most common causes of bronchiectasis are severe parenchymal infections of the lung, including pertussis and measles in childhood and, most importantly in the developing world, tuberculosis (Table 5.1).

Pathogenesis. The initial feature is damage to the conducting airways of the lung and interference with mucociliary clearance. Once bronchiectasis is present, repeated infections serve to maintain a vicious cycle of inflammation and damage to the already compromised airway, which leads to further

TABLE 5.1

Common causes of bronchiectasis

- Childhood infections including pertussis and measles
- Tuberculosis
- Foreign bodies
- Carcinoma
- Allergic bronchopulmonary aspergillosis (ABPA)
- Rheumatoid disease
- Immunoglobulin deficiency (including subclass deficiency, particularly IgG_2, IgG_4)
- Ciliary abnormalities (e.g. Kartagener's syndrome)
- Cystic fibrosis

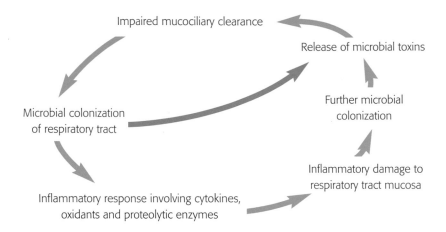

Figure 5.1 Vicious circle hypothesis of pathogenesis of bronchiectasis. Adapted from Cole PJ, Wilson R. Host–microbial interrelationships in respiratory infection. *Chest* 1989;95:2175–83.

infection (Figure 5.1). The sputum of patients with bronchiectasis is chronically infected with the following pathogens:

- *H. influenzae*
- *S. pneumoniae*
- *S. aureus*
- *P. aeruginosa*.

Extracellular products of each of these organisms are capable of exacerbating the disruption in mucociliary clearance, either by a direct effect on the epithelial cells of the airway, or by induction of an inflammatory infiltrate. In established disease, chronic infection with *P. aeruginosa* is associated with a particularly poor prognosis.

Clinical features. The most prominent clinical feature of bronchiectasis is a cough that produces large quantities (e.g. a cupful per day) of purulent phlegm (which, on standing, shows characteristic sputum layering), together with fatigue and wheeze. During exacerbations, patients may be breathless, wheezy and febrile. In severe cases, clubbing is present.

Diagnosis is usually clinically obvious in patients with extensive bronchiectasis, but in patients with relatively minor, focal disease, the

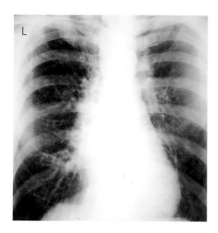

Figure 5.2 A chest radiograph from a patient with Kartagener's syndrome ('L' indicates the left side of the patient's chest). The patient demonstrated situs inversus with dextrocardia. The lung fields show tramlines and ring shadows. Reproduced courtesy of Dr R Peck, Royal Hallamshire Hospital, Sheffield, UK.

diagnosis may be suggested by recurrent lower respiratory tract infections that are slow to clear. The diagnosis is essentially radiological.
The chest radiograph may be normal, or demonstrate abnormal thick, dilated bronchi producing ring shadows or tramlines (Figure 5.2). High-resolution CT scanning of the thorax may demonstrate dilated airways and bronchial wall thickening (Figure 5.3).

In patients with newly diagnosed bronchiectasis, a number of investigations may elucidate the cause. These include:

- immunoglobulins, including subclasses (total immunoglobulin can be normal in patients with a subclass deficiency)
- rheumatoid factor

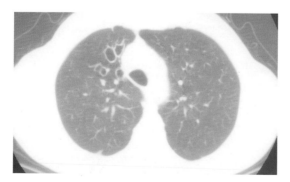

Figure 5.3 High-resolution CT scan showing grossly dilated airways with bronchial wall thickening in a patient with bronchiectasis. Reproduced with permission from Dr R Nakielny, Royal Hallamshire Hospital, Sheffield, UK.

- *Aspergillus* precipitins
- microscopy/EM studies to identify ciliary abnormalities.

The distribution of the bronchiectasis is related to the initiating cause. In general, bronchiectasis resulting from a generalized abnormality, such as a ciliary abnormality, cystic fibrosis or hypogammaglobulinaemia, is widespread and affects both the proximal and distal airways. In contrast, bronchiectasis resulting from tuberculosis or impaction of a foreign body is usually localized to a lobe or bronchopulmonary segment; upper lobe involvement is particularly common following allergic bronchopulmonary aspergillosis and tuberculosis.

During exacerbations, sputum should always be sent to the laboratory for microbiological examination to determine antibiotic susceptibilities and, in particular, to identify infection with beta-lactamase-secreting *H. influenza*e and also *P. aeruginosa*, both of which are unlikely to respond to aminopenicillins.

Management. The mainstay of treatment of bronchiectasis is drainage, which can be provided by a combination of postural drainage (Figure 5.4) and physiotherapy. These measures reduce the frequency of exacerbations and the need for antibiotic therapy if conducted on a daily basis.

Antibiotic therapy. Beta-lactams do not penetrate bronchiectatic tissue well at conventional doses, but high doses of amoxycillin (e.g. 6 g/day) are more effective in terminating exacerbations. High doses of oral cephalosporins or ciprofloxacin are also effective when beta-lactamase-producing strains are isolated. In out-patients colonized with *P. aeruginosa*,

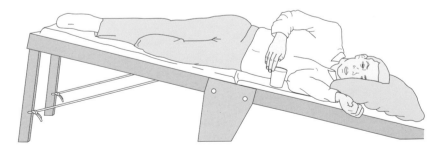

Figure 5.4 Postural drainage in the management of bronchiectasis. The patient is tipped at an angle of approximately 20°.

intermittent use of high-dose oral ciprofloxacin for exacerbations is the mainstay of therapy.

Long-term oral antibiotics are well tolerated and can lead to symptomatic improvement, but ciprofloxacin-resistant *P. aeruginosa* may be troublesome. The use of a prophylactic aminoglycoside given by nebulizer (e.g. nebulized gentamicin) is of dubious value, but there are numerous anecdotal reports of success.

In extremely severe exacerbations requiring hospitalization, an intravenous antibiotic effective against *H. influenzae* and *P. aeruginosa* (e.g. ceftazidime, aminoglycosides or ciprofloxacin) is indicated.

Surgery. Surgical excision of bronchiectatic tissue was widely used in the past, particularly in patients with localized disease. Nowadays, however, it is seldom performed, because thin-cut CT scanning has shown that most patients have widespread disease to some extent. In patients with extremely severe bronchiectasis that is life-threatening, heart–lung transplantation may be indicated.

Cystic fibrosis

Cystic fibrosis is an autosomal recessive disease resulting from a mutation of the cystic fibrosis gene on chromosome 7. Approximately 5% of Caucasians carry the gene, and about 6000 people in the UK and 30 000 in the USA are affected. The mutation results in absence or poor functioning of the cystic fibrosis transmembrane regulator (CFTR) protein. This leads to pancreatic dysfunction and an associated abnormality of airway secretions, in which mucins form thick gels altering their rheological properties. The resulting thick tenacious sputum in the airways causes obstruction leading to recurrent infection.

Clinical features. Infants present with:
- meconium ileus at birth
- diarrhoea or malabsorption in infancy
- failure to thrive
- progressive cough
- recurrent pneumonia.

Pulmonary disease may, in some cases, be relatively mild or even present for the first time in adult life. In most young children with moderately severe

51

disease, acute exacerbations occur with increased sputum production, cyanosis, dyspnoea, fever and weight loss. Patients also suffer from nasal polyposis and chronic sinusitis.

Microbiology. The first pathogen to colonize children with cystic fibrosis is *S. aureus*. Exotoxins of *S. aureus* induce bronchial wall injury and abscess formation. The intense inflammatory response to *S. aureus* ultimately leads to tissue destruction and bronchiectasis.

The defect in mucociliary clearance in these patients, together with injury due to staphylococcal infections permits colonization by other bacteria including *P. aeruginosa*. Patients are at first colonized by non-mucoid strains, but later, mucoid variants emerge. These strains cannot be completely eradicated, despite the high antibody levels observed in patients, and the intensive antibiotic therapy that they receive. Once *P. aeruginosa* infection is established, it is impossible to eradicate, and bacterial proteases produced by the bacteria cause significant damage to the airways. *P. aeruginosa* pigments interfere with mucociliary function. Other products, including the haemolysin rhamnolipid, also reduce mucociliary transport.

Other organisms often isolated from the sputum of cystic fibrosis patients include non-typable *H. influenzae* and *S. pneumoniae*. *Burkholderia cepacia* also colonizes these patients and is transmissible between close contacts. This organism can occasionally be responsible for a fulminating septicaemia. It is intrinsically highly resistant to antibiotics including those effective against *P. aeruginosa*, but is usually sensitive to trimethoprim–sulphamethoxazole and chloramphenicol. A range of other bacteria, including the Enterobacteriaceae and *Stenotrephomonas (xanthomonas) maltophilia,* can also colonize such patients. In patients with severe disease, *Candida albicans, Aspergillus* and environmental mycobacteria can also occasionally be isolated in the sputum.

Diagnosis. The diagnosis rests on the clinical presentation, nasal potential difference and sweat chloride concentrations, and can be confirmed by genotyping. A sweat chloride concentration of over 70 mEq/litre usually indicates cystic fibrosis. In adults, such investigations may be prompted by recurrent pneumonias or by unexplained isolation of *P. aeruginosa* from an adolescent or an adult with bronchiectasis.

Management. Daily postural drainage and physiotherapy are mandatory in patients with established bronchiectasis due to cystic fibrosis. Once disease is established, some physicians attempt to suppress sputum colonization by long-term administration of antibiotics including:

- oral cephalosporins
- oral chloramphenicol
- trimethoprim–sulphamethoxazole
- co-amoxiclav.

However, such an approach has not been proved to be effective. Most centres treat only acute exacerbations of pulmonary infection, with inclusion of empirical anti-*Pseudomonas* and anti-*S. aureus* antibiotics. Appropriate intravenous therapy might include:

- a beta-lactam plus an aminoglycoside
- ceftazidime plus an aminoglycoside
- ciprofloxacin
- an anti-*Pseudomonas* penicillin plus aminoglycoside
- an anti-*Pseudomonas* penicillin with a beta-lactamase inhibitor.

In principle, antibiotic regimens should be rotated, and directed by sputum evaluation and microbial sensitivities.

Intravenous therapy administered at home is now widely used in these patients and appropriate antibiotics include ceftazidime, the penems, monobactams, and beta-lactam–beta-lactamase inhibitors. Unfortunately, monotherapy can result in the spread of resistant organisms (e.g. *P. aeruginosa*), particularly with the use of ceftazidime, imipenem and aztreonam.

Oral quinolones, such as ciprofloxacin, have permitted more flexible management of exacerbations and are now routinely used in children with cystic fibrosis in most centres. Although resistant *P. aeruginosa* can emerge during therapy with ciprofloxacin, *in-vitro* susceptibility of isolates returns when the quinolones are withheld for 3 months. Nebulized antibiotics, including tobramycin, have been shown to eradicate *P. aeruginosa*, but emergence of resistant strains during therapy has been a problem.

Other modes of therapy under evaluation include DNAase, which reduces sputum viscosity, and amiloride and triphosphate nucleotides, which restore salt and water secretions.

CHAPTER 6

Pneumonia in the immunocompromised host

Pulmonary disease in an immunocompromised host may be due to a number of infectious or non-infectious causes that can each occur with or without fever.

Non-infectious causes

Non-infectious causes of pulmonary infiltrates include:

- pulmonary oedema
- cytotoxic drug-induced lung injury (e.g. bleomycin injury)
- pulmonary haemorrhage
- radiation pneumonitis
- pulmonary infiltration of the underlying malignancy
- organizing pneumonitis.

Large-volume infusions of chemotherapeutic agents can lead to pulmonary oedema, particularly in severely ill or septic patients with impaired renal function or other factors that increase susceptibility to this condition. Interstitial lung injury induced by cytotoxic drugs (e.g. bleomycin) is usually most severe after cumulative doses of 150 mg or more, but can occur at lower doses following combination chemotherapy.

Radiation pneumonitis usually occurs at least 1 month after irradiation, in a pattern that exactly traces the therapeutic field. Infiltrative malignancies (e.g. lymphangitic carcinomatosis, non-Hodgkin's lymphoma) are generally insidious and evidence of malignant spread elsewhere (for instance, to the liver or bone) may be seen.

Infectious causes

In general, susceptibility to infection can be classified according to the underlying defect of innate or specific-acquired immunity. Extracellular pathogens, such as certain bacteria or fungi, are able to flourish in patients with functional defects in complement, antibodies or phagocytes (e.g. neutrophils or macrophages). Defence against intracellular pathogens requires efficient activity of T-helper cells or cytotoxic T cells. Infections associated with specific common defects of the inflammatory or immunological response are shown in Table 6.1.

TABLE 6.1

Infections associated with common defects in inflammatory or immunological responses

Host defect	Examples of diseases associated with defect	Common infections
Neutropenia	• Haematological malignancies • Cytotoxic chemotherapy	• Gram-negative bacillary pneumonia • *Staphylococcus aureus* pneumonia • Invasive *Aspergillus* infection
Ineffective macrophage phagocytosis	• Systemic lupus erythematosus (SLE) • Diabetes • Non-Hodgkin's leukaemia	Pneumonia due to: • *Streptococcus pneumoniae* • *Haemophilus influenzae* • *Staphylococcus aureus*
Complement deficiency	• SLE • Congenital deficiency	Pneumonia due to: • *Streptococcus pneumoniae* • *Pseudomonas* spp.
Antibody deficiency	• Hypogammaglobulinaemia • Multiple myeloma • Chronic lymphocytic leukaemia	Pneumonia due to: • *Streptococcus pneumoniae* • *Haemophilus influenzae* • *Staphylococcus aureus* • *Klebsiella* spp. • Gram-negative bacilli
T-lymphocyte deficiency/ dysfunction	• Hodgkin's disease • AIDS • Organ transplantation • High-dose corticosteroid therapy	• *Pneumocystis carinii* • Cytomegalovirus • Herpes simplex virus • *Mycobacterium* spp. • *Aspergillus* spp. • *Cryptococcus neoformans* • *Legionella* spp. • *Nocardia* spp.

Clinical features

Patients with an infective pneumonitis usually have fever together with cough and dyspnoea.

Time course of illness. Individual infections vary in their severity and speed of evolution. In AIDS, *Pneumocystis carinii* pneumonia (PCP) has an indolent course with symptoms extending over 3–4 weeks. In contrast, PCP in patients with other immunocompromising disorders (e.g. Hodgkin's disease) is acute and fulminant. Similarly, bacterial infections are rapid and aggressive, particularly in the neutropenic host. Some infections evolve over 1–2 weeks; these include cytomegalovirus (CMV), pneumonitis in organ transplant patients, *Aspergillus* infections in neutropenic patients, and cryptococcosis in patients with AIDS. Mycobacterial infections and other chronic bacterial infections (e.g. *Nocardia*) tend to evolve slowly.

Degree of immunosuppression. Pneumonitis in neutropenic patients tends to occur when the absolute neutrophil count is less than 0.5×10^9/litre. In AIDS patients, pneumonitis due to *P. carinii* or *Cryptococcus neoformans* is generally seen when the CD4 count falls below 0.2×10^9/litre, and *Mycobacterium intracellulare* disease when the CD4 count falls below 0.05×10^9/litre.

Time of onset. In organ transplant recipients, CMV pneumonia tends to occur 1–6 months after surgery, and does not occur before or after this period.

Physical examination of the chest may be normal even when the chest radiograph reveals extensive infiltration. A number of features may, however, be helpful in the assessment of aetiology and severity of pneumonitis.
- Respiratory rate is a sensitive marker of severity.
- Subtle features (e.g. rales) may become apparent before the chest radiograph becomes abnormal.
- The presence of localized wheeze may indicate a partially obstructed bronchus, suggestive of neoplastic infiltration.
- The presence of a pleural rub in an aggressive pneumonitis suggests bacterial or *Aspergillus* infection, but is seldom present in PCP.

Chest radiographs may reveal characteristic features (Figure 6.1; Table 6.2).

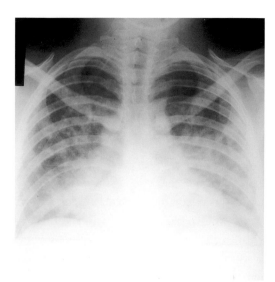

Figure 6.1 This patient presented 6 weeks after renal transplant with high fever and dry cough. Immunofluorescence of bronchoalveolar lavage was positive for cytomegalovirus, and transbronchial biopsy revealed cells with 'owls-eye' inclusion bodies typical of cytomegalovirus infection.

TABLE 6.2

Characteristic radiographic features of pulmonary disease in the immunocompromised host

Diffuse infiltrates

- *Pneumocystis carinii* pneumonia (PCP)
- Cytomegalovirus pneumonitis
- Pulmonary oedema
- Lymphangitic carcinomatosis

Nodular or cavitating lesions

- Mycobacterial infections
- Cryptococcal infections
- *Nocardia* infections
- Invasive *Aspergillus* infection

Focal infiltrates

- Bacterial pneumonias
- *Cryptococcus neoformans*
- Radiation pneumonitis
- Invasive *Aspergillus* infection

Laboratory diagnosis

In general, samples should be taken for laboratory diagnosis in parallel with the institution of empirical therapy. Sputum and blood culture will yield a diagnosis in a small number of patients. Serology for CMV, cryptococcal antigen or *L. pneumophila* is relatively unhelpful in the acute phase of the illness.

The following lung-sampling or biopsy techniques are the most useful for diagnosis.

- Induced sputum using 3% nebulized saline can reveal a diagnosis in patients with diffuse infiltrates on the chest radiograph, particularly in patients with AIDS. This technique may reveal infection with *P. carinii* or *Mycobacteria*.
- Bronchoalveolar lavage has a sensitivity of greater than 90% in detecting PCP in patients with AIDS and a sensitivity of 40–80% in patients with other immunocompromising illnesses.
- Transbronchial biopsy can be conducted at the same time as bronchoalveolar lavage. It is particularly useful in the diagnosis of diffuse pulmonary infiltrates due to infection.
- Open lung biopsy is the gold standard for diagnosis and provides a diagnosis in more than 90% of patients.

Techniques. Sputum and bronchial washings can be subjected to the following staining techniques:

- Gram stain to identify conventional pathogens
- Ziehl-Neelsen stain to identify *Mycobacteria* and *Nocardia*
- india ink to identify *Cryptococcus*
- potassium hydroxide to identify *Aspergillus* and *Mucor*
- methenamine silver stain to identify *P. carinii*
- Wright-Giemsa stain to identify CMV
- monoclonal antibodies (direct immunofluorescence) to identify *Legionella*, *P. carinii*, CMV and herpes simplex virus.

Culture techniques include:

- blood/lysed blood agar to identify conventional pathogens
- Lowenstein-Jensen to identify *Mycobacterium* spp.
- Sabouraud agar to identify *Mucor*, *Candida*, *Nocardia* and *Cryptococcus*
- cell culture to identify CMV and herpes simplex virus.

PNEUMONIA IN THE IMMUNOCOMPROMISED HOST

Management

Unfortunately, the low yield of non-invasive investigations, and the frailty of patients often necessitates a full empirical approach. An organized strategy has been suggested by Fanta and Pennington (Figure 6.2).

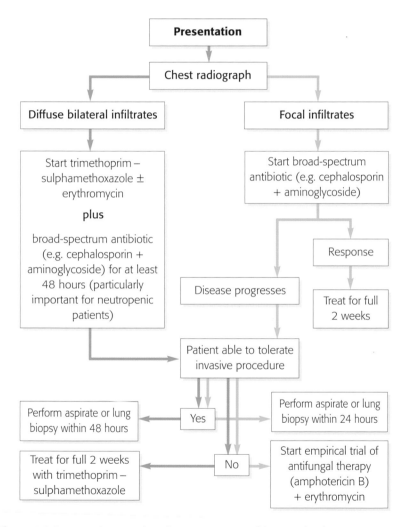

Figure 6.2 Suggested approach to the management of fever and pulmonary infiltrates in the immunocompromised host. Adapted with permission from Pennington JE, ed. Fanta CH, Pennington JE. In: *Respiratory Infections. Diagnosis and Management.* Third edition. New York: Raven Press, 1994.

In patients with focal infiltrates, particularly neutropenic patients, antibiotic cover against Gram-negative bacilli (including *P. aeruginosa*) and *Staphylococci* is necessary. Suitable combinations include:

- a third-generation cephalosporin (e.g. ceftazidime) plus an aminoglycoside
- a broad-spectrum penicillin (e.g. ticarcillin or piperacillin) plus an aminoglycoside plus a glycopeptide (e.g. vancomycin)
- piperacillin/tazobactam plus ciprofloxacin.

In patients who have bilateral pulmonary infiltrates, particularly those with a type of immunosuppression that generally favours overgrowth with *P. carinii*, empirical therapy with trimethoprim–sulphamethoxazole is warranted, together with therapy directed against *L. pneumophila*, which commonly presents with bilateral infiltrates.

Every effort should be made to make a diagnosis by either induction of sputum, bronchoalveolar lavage or lung biopsy in order to spare the patient 2 weeks of unnecessary therapy; in some centres, however, it is common practice to wait and see whether there is a response to empirical therapy before employing invasive diagnostic techniques.

The clinical condition of some patients with localized infiltrates is too severe to warrant invasive diagnostic techniques. If these patients fail to respond to initial empirical antimicrobial therapy, an alternative choice is to initiate erythromycin together with empirical antifungal therapy (amphotericin B).

CHAPTER 7

HIV infection and pulmonary disease

The lung is an important site of disease in patients with HIV infection. Pulmonary complications can occur at any stage of the illness (Figure 7.1; Table 7.1).

In developed countries, the most common problems involving the lung are acute bronchitis, pneumococcal pneumonia and PCP. In general, pulmonary complications are related to the immune status (CD4 count) and the risk factor associated with HIV infection for each individual. In the USA, the Pulmonary Complications of HIV Infection Study has shown that most individuals with early HIV disease experience relatively minor respiratory problems, including upper respiratory tract infections (e.g. sinusitis and acute bronchitis). Those with CD4 counts between 0.2×10^9/litre and 0.5×10^9/litre are at increased risk of developing PCP and bacterial pneumonia, especially

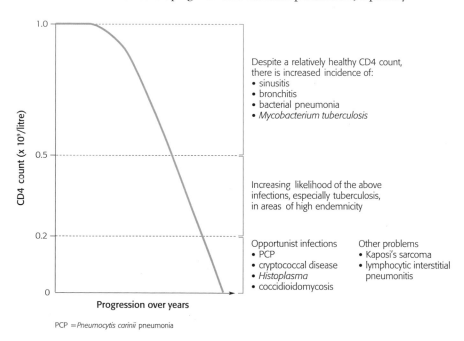

PCP = *Pneumocytis carinii* pneumonia

Figure 7.1 Relationship between the natural history of HIV infection and pulmonary complications.

TABLE 7.1

Pulmonary complications in HIV infection

Bacteria

- *Mycobacterium tuberculosis*
- *Mycobacterium kansasii*
- *Mycobacterium avium* complex
- *Streptococcus pneumoniae*
- *Haemophilus influenzae*
- *Staphylococcus aureus*
- *Moraxella catarrhalis*
- *Pseudomonas aeruginosa*
- *Nocardia asteroides*
- *Rhodococcus equi*

Lung tumours

- Kaposi's sarcoma
- Non-Hodgkin's lymphoma

Fungal infection

- *Pneumocystis carinii*
- *Cryptococcus neoformans*
- *Histoplasma capsulatum*
- *Coccidioides immitis*
- *Aspergillus fumigatus*
- *Penicillium marneffei*

Viruses

- Cytomegalovirus
- Herpes simplex virus

Lymphocytic interstitial pneumonitis

S. pneumoniae. In severely immunocompromised patients (CD4 < 0.2×10^9/litre), PCP and bacterial pneumonia occur at much higher rates, even when chemoprophylaxis (e.g. trimethoprim–sulphamethoxazole) is used. It remains to be seen how highly active antiretroviral therapy (HAART) will influence pulmonary disease over the next few years, but a marked reduction in the incidence of PCP is currently being observed.

Diagnosis

The CD4 count is an important guide in the evaluation of patients with pulmonary symptoms and signs. However, the clinical history together with a few simple investigations can usually establish the diagnosis (Figure 7.2). The relevant clinical features that may help to distinguish the more common pulmonary complications are listed in Table 7.2.

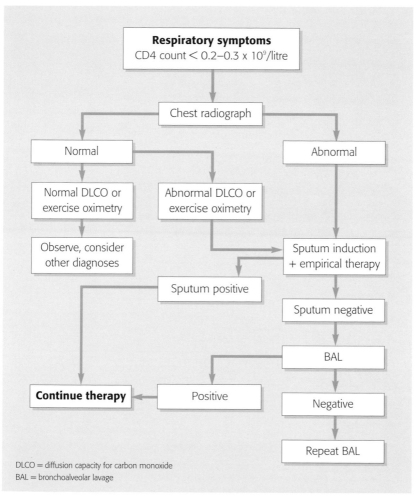

Figure 7.2 Approach to pulmonary symptoms in patients with HIV infection.

Investigations. An initial chest radiograph may provide important diagnostic clues (Table 7.3; Figures 7.3 and 7.4). In patients with normal chest radiographs, indicators of significant pulmonary disease include:

- a carbon monoxide diffusion capacity less than 80% of predicted value
- uptake on Gallium lung scanning
- a greater than 5% drop in oxygen saturation on exercise oximetry.

Respiratory secretions can be obtained either by induction of sputum production using ultrasonic nebulization of 3% saline, or by

TABLE 7.2

Characteristic clinical features of common pulmonary complications

Pneumocystis carinii pneumonia

- Absence of prophylaxis
- Insidious onset
- Prodrome of fevers, night sweats, weight loss and oral candidiasis
- Dry cough
- Retrosternal irritation on deep breath
- Absence of pleuritic chest pain
- CD4 count < 0.2 x 10^9/litre
- Reduced carbon monoxide diffusion capacity

Bacterial pneumonia

- Severe and abrupt onset
- Productive cough
- Pleuritic chest pain
- High peripheral white blood cell count

Tuberculosis

Early disease

- Cough with or without haemoptysis
- Weight loss
- Localized or diffuse lung abnormalities on the chest radiograph

Late disease

- Pronounced constitutional symptoms
- Diffuse infiltrates on the chest radiograph

Kaposi's sarcoma

- Insidious onset of dyspnoea
- Persistent cough
- Presence of lesions elsewhere

Fungal diseases (*Histoplasma, Coccidioides*)

- Residence in endemic area

HIV INFECTION AND PULMONARY DISEASE

TABLE 7.3

Characteristic findings on the chest radiograph in common pulmonary complications of HIV infection

Characteristic finding	Possible diagnosis
Normal	• *Pneumocystis carinii* pneumonia • Disseminated fungal infection
Focal infiltrate	• Bacterial pneumonia • *Mycobacterium tuberculosis* • Fungal pneumonia • *Pneumocystis carinii* pneumonia
Pleural effusion	• Kaposi's sarcoma • Bacterial pneumonia • *Mycobacterium tuberculosis*
Hilar lymphadenopathy	• *Mycobacterium tuberculosis* • Lymphoma
Interstitial infiltrate	• *Pneumocystis carinii* pneumonia • *Mycobacterium tuberculosis* • Lymphocytic interstitial pneumonitis • Bacterial pneumonia

bronchoalveolar lavage. The secretions should be examined by:

- microbiological staining for *P. carinii* (e.g. modified Giemsa, methenamine silver, toluidine blue O)
- Ziehl-Neelsen or auramine staining for *Mycobacteria*
- culture for *Mycobacteria*, other bacteria, fungi and viruses
- monoclonal antibody-based immunofluorescence assays for *P. carinii*, herpes simplex virus, CMV and *L. pneumophila*.

Although sputum induction is a valuable investigation, its negative predictive value is relatively poor; thus, patients with a negative induced sputum result should undergo fibre-optic bronchoscopy.

The combination of bronchoalveolar lavage and transbronchial biopsy will yield a diagnosis in more than 95% of lower respiratory tract infections in patients with AIDS.

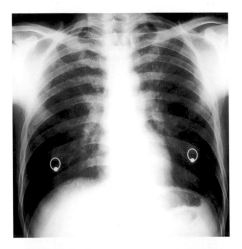

Figure 7.3 This patient presented with a 4-week history of night sweats and dry cough. The chest radiograph shows diffuse bilateral infiltrates. Induced sputum was positive for *Pneumocystis carinii,* and the patient tested positive for HIV antibody. Reproduced courtesy of Dr R Peck, Royal Hallamshire Hospital, Sheffield, UK.

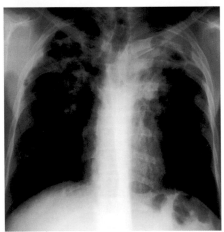

Figure 7.4 This HIV-positive patient presented with 1 month of productive cough and weight loss. The chest radiograph revealed extensive nodular and cavitating consolidation of both upper lobes. Auramine stain of sputum revealed acid-fast bacilli, and culture revealed multi-drug resistant *Mycobacterium tuberculosis*.

Treatment of *Pneumocystis carinii* pneumonia

A number of therapeutic options are available depending on the severity of the disease (Table 7.4); the adjunctive use of corticosteroids in patients with *P. carinii* infection is now well established.

Prevention of pulmonary complications

Pneumocystis carinii infection. All patients with a CD4 count below 0.2×10^9/litre should be offered prophylaxis against *P. carinii*. A major problem is intolerance of some regimens, particularly those involving trimethoprim–sulphamethoxazole. However, a wide range of drugs is

TABLE 7.4

Treatment of *Pneumocystis carinii* pneumonia

Disease status	Recommended therapy	Alternative therapy	Comments
Mild disease (patient ambulant, $PaO_2 > 8$ kPa)	Trimethoprim, 20 mg/kg/day PLUS sulphamethoxazole, oral, 100 mg/kg every 12 hours for 21 days	Dapsone, oral, 100 mg daily, plus trimethoprim, oral, 5 mg/kg every 8 hours	If rash due to trimethoprim– sulphamethoxazole occurs, dose can be reduced to trimethoprim, 15 mg/kg/day, plus sulphamethoxazole, 75 mg/kg/day
		Atovaquone, oral, 750 mg every 8 hours	
		Clindamycin, 450 mg every 6 hours, plus primaquine, oral, 15 mg daily	Clindamycin plus primaquine is highly effective, but often causes severe rash and diarrhoea
Moderate– severe disease ($PaO_2 < 8$ kPa)	Trimethoprim, 20 mg/kg/day, plus sulphamethoxazole, i.v., 100 mg/kg/day PLUS prednisolone, oral, 40 mg every 12 hours or hydrocortisone, 200 mg, i.v., every 6 hours for 5 days, gradually reducing dose over 21 days	Pentamidine, i.v., 4 mg/kg every 24 hours	Pentamidine is toxic (rashes, hypoglycaemia, renal dysfunction), but is the most potent alternative to trimethoprim– sulphamethoxazole
		Clindamycin, i.v., 600 mg every 6 hours, plus primaquine, oral, 15–30 mg daily	
		Trimetrexate, i.v., 45 mg/m² every 24 hours, plus leucovorin, i.v., 20 mg/m² every 6 hours	Trimetrexate is well tolerated, but not as effective as trimethoprim– sulphamethoxazole

available and a suitable regimen can usually be tailored for each patient (Table 7.5). Nevertheless, trimethoprim–sulphamethoxazole has been the most successful therapy, and breakthrough infections are more commonly seen with aerosolized pentamidine or dapsone.

TABLE 7.5

Prophylaxis for HIV-related opportunistic infections

Pathogen	Indication for prophylaxis	First choice
Pneumocystis carinii	CD4 count < 0.2 x 10^9/litre Persistent unexplained fever Chronic oropharyngeal candidiasis	Trimethoprim (80–160 mg)–sulphamethoxazole (400–800 mg), oral, daily Dapsone, 100 mg, daily
Mycobacterium tuberculosis	Tuberculin test positive (> 5 mm)	Isoniazid, 300 mg, daily for 12 months
Pneumococcus	All patients	Pneumovax
Haemophilus influenzae	No consensus	Hib vaccine
Influenza	All patients	Influenza vaccine

Streptococcus pneumoniae. Use of the 23-valent polysaccharide vaccine has been evaluated in patients with HIV. Clinical efficacy is impaired in patients with advanced disease, but the vaccine should be routinely offered to new patients, particularly those with early disease.

Mycobacterium tuberculosis. Tuberculin testing should be offered to all patients with HIV infection, but BCG vaccination is absolutely contraindicated. In patients who convert their tuberculin skin test, prophylaxis with isoniazid, 300 mg/day, should be offered.

Alternatives	Comments
Aerosolized pentamidine Dapsone, 100 mg plus pyrimethamine, 25 mg, once weekly	Aerosolized pentamidine should be delivered by Respirgard II® or Fisoneb® nebulizer Trimethoprim–sulphamethoxazole can probably be given 2 or 3 days weekly with high efficacy; single-strength tablets are also effective
	In patients exposed to resistant strains, two-drug regimens, using combinations of rifampicin, pyrazinamide or a quinolone, can be considered
	Trimethoprim–sulphamethoxazole appears to prevent some disease
	Trimethoprim–sulphamethoxazole appears to prevent some disease

CHAPTER 8

Viral pneumonias

Influenza

Pneumonia due to influenza virus infection is most commonly seen in adults. Winter epidemics of influenza A and influenza B occur worldwide. Currently, the H1N1 and H3N2 subtypes are responsible for most epidemics of influenza A, though in the latter half of 1997, an outbreak of an avian subtype H5N1 was reported in Hong Kong.

Clinical features. Lower respiratory tract symptoms of pneumonia typically follow 24 hours after the typical 'flu' symptoms with high fever, increasing dyspnoea and wheezing. Haemoptysis may be present. The chest radiograph usually shows a diffuse non-lobar infiltrate. Bacterial superinfection of viral pneumonia may occur either simultaneously with the viral pneumonitis or a few days following the initial illness. The bacteria most commonly implicated in such superinfections are *S. pneumoniae*, *S. aureus* and *H. influenzae*.

Diagnosis. The gold standard for diagnosis is culture of virus respiratory secretions, which are most efficiently obtained by nasopharyngeal aspiration (Figure 8.1). Culture on MDCK or Vero cells generally takes 7–14 days. Rapid diagnostic techniques, such as rapid culture, direct immuno-fluorescence (which has reduced sensitivity) and PCR tests are currently being adopted as routine laboratory tests.

Figure 8.1
Nasopharyngeal aspiration.

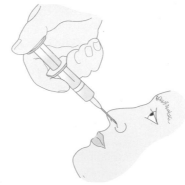

Treatment. Amantadine hydrochloride is useful for prophylaxis against influenza A infections, but is ineffective against influenza B. In hospital personnel exposed to influenza virus, amantadine hydrochloride has been shown to have an efficacy of approximately 60% in preventing clinical disease. Some small studies have also demonstrated improvement in symptoms in established pneumonia.

Prevention. Influenza vaccine is generally administered to elderly patients or those with chronic lung disease. It is a killed vaccine composed of the predicted subtypes for each annual season.

Respiratory syncytial virus

Respiratory syncytial virus (RSV) is the most common cause of viral pneumonia in children aged 6 months to 3 years in the UK and the USA. It is highly infectious, and spreads rapidly within hospitals and child-care facilities.

Clinical features. Infection can result in bronchiolitis and pneumonia, with prominent wheezing on auscultation and pulmonary infiltrates on the chest radiograph. The disease can be severe in children receiving cytotoxic chemotherapy for malignant disease; however, corticosteroids appear to have no effect on disease severity.

Diagnosis. The diagnosis can rapidly be made by immunofluorescence of nasopharyngeal aspirates (Figure 8.2) or by culture, which generally takes between 7 and 10 days.

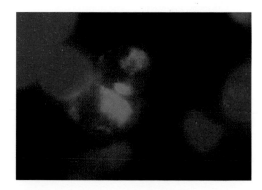

Figure 8.2 Immunofluorescence of nasopharyngeal aspirate from a patient with RSV infection.

Treatment and prevention. Aerosolized ribavirin is used routinely to treat severe RSV pneumonia in infants and children. Infants treated with ribavirin demonstrate more rapid normalization of blood gases and reduction in viral shedding. Hyperimmune RSV immunoglobulin is available in the USA for prophylaxis in high-risk infants.

Adenovirus

In most cases, adenovirus pneumonia is caused by serotypes 4, 7 or 21. It occurs both in children and in adults.

Clinical features. Although adenovirus is a common cause of conjunctivitis, this is usually absent in patients with pneumonia. Rather there is gradual onset of illness consisting of fever, dry cough and dyspnoea. Occasionally, pleural effusions and rhabdomyolysis are seen in children but the mortality is very low. Bronchiectasis is a well-documented sequel of childhood adenovirus pneumonia.

Diagnosis is usually either by culture of respiratory secretions or serology. Some centres offer direct immunofluorescence of respiratory secretions.

Treatment. No specific therapy for adenovirus pneumonia has been developed.

Measles

Although respiratory symptoms are fairly common in measles, pneumonia with the appearance of pulmonary infiltrates on the chest radiograph is thought to occur in less than 5% of cases in the developed world; it is much more common in developing countries, where it has been linked to vitamin A deficiency. In most cases, a fine reticular nodular infiltrate can be seen on the chest radiograph. Measles pneumonia can be severe, particularly in malnourished children, in immunocompromised patients and in pregnant women.

Diagnosis can be made by detection of salivary IgM, or by culture of virus from saliva.

Prevention. The incidence of measles and the associated pneumonia has been
dramatically reduced by the use of the live attenuated measles vaccine,

which is usually given as part of the MMR (measles, mumps and rubella) vaccination shortly after the first birthday and before school entry in the UK.

Treatment is generally supportive or aimed at control of bacterial superinfection.

Varicella zoster virus pneumonia

Chickenpox can be complicated by pneumonia in approximately 10–20% of cases in adults, but is rare in children. It is more common in adults who smoke. Pneumonia usually occurs in those patients with the most severe skin rash and can be severe, particularly in immunocompromised patients and in pregnant women.

Clinical features. Patients with varicella zoster virus (VZV) pneumonia may have a dry cough and dyspnoea, and crackles can often be heard on auscultation. The chest radiograph shows a fine nodular infiltrate (Figure 8.3), which calcifies over many years to leave punctate diffuse pulmonary calcification scattered widely throughout the lung fields.

Diagnosis. Chest radiographs should be routinely taken for patients with chickenpox and respiratory signs or symptoms, and digital pulse oximetry should be performed.

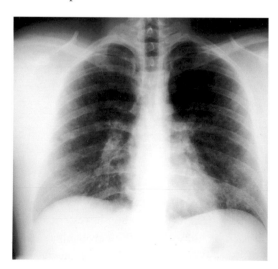

Figure 8.3 The fine nodular infiltrate that develops during varicella zoster virus pneumonia. This calcifies over many years to leave punctate diffuse pulmonary calcification scattered widely throughout the lung fields.

Prevention. A live attenuated VZV vaccine has been developed and is currently being evaluated in the developed world.

Treatment. Acyclovir, 5–10 mg/kg, i.v., three times/day, should be administered to patients with VZV pneumonitis. The drug is well tolerated and can be used in pregnancy. Clear benefit has been shown only when the drug has been administered within 48 hours of the onset of the rash.

Cytomegalovirus

CMV pneumonitis is nearly always seen in immunocompromised patients, particularly those who are immunocompromised as part of bone marrow or renal transplant procedures. CMV pneumonitis may be seen in late-stage AIDS, usually in the context of co-existent *P. carinii* infection.

Clinical features. CMV pneumonitis usually occurs as part of a systemic syndrome, with hepatitis or involvement of the gastrointestinal tract. Patients complain of fever and other systemic symptoms, together with dry cough and dyspnoea. The chest radiograph reveals a diffuse interstitial pneumonitis. The illness can be extremely severe and fatal.

Diagnosis is most easily made in patients who have previously been seronegative for CMV and who become seropositive during their acute illness. Culture of the virus from respiratory secretions or the demonstration of the virus by direct immunofluorescence may also aid diagnosis. Lung biopsy may reveal focal areas of inflammatory infiltration including cytomegaly, with 'owls-eye' inclusions.

Treatment. Ganciclovir, particularly in combination with intravenous immunoglobulin, has improved the prognosis in patients with CMV pneumonitis.

Hantavirus

Hantavirus infection emerged during the 1990s as a cause of severe respiratory illness. The illness has been described in the South-western USA, particularly among American Indians. Hantavirus infection probably results from contact with the deer-mouse, but other rodents may also be involved.

Clinical features comprise sudden onset of fever and headache, and some systemic symptoms, together with a rapidly progressing respiratory illness usually beginning with dry cough. The chest radiograph demonstrates features consistent with adult respiratory distress syndrome. The disease has a high mortality, possibly as great as 50%.

Diagnosis. Antibodies to hantavirus can be detected by ELISA.

Prevention. Rodent control programmes should be initiated in areas with outbreaks of hantavirus infection.

Treatment. Intravenous ribavirin has been used successfully in patients with severe hantavirus pneumonitis.

CHAPTER 9

Future trends

In addressing 'future trends' in this field, it is tempting to launch immediately into discussions of molecular-genetic-based diagnostics, second-generation fluoroquinolones, and the impact of highly active antiretroviral treatment on lung infections in patients with AIDS. However, first it is important to remind ourselves that the foundation for major advances in our understanding of respiratory tract infections has been, is, and will be, careful clinical observation. Modern trends in diagnosis and therapy are the direct result of strategies based on key clinical observations in the past.

Numerous examples exist of important lessons learned by 'old-fashioned' clinical deduction while caring for patients with respiratory infection. However, a few key lessons deserve to be singled out. These observations include the description of non-pneumococcal bacterial community-acquired pneumonias in certain types of hosts (1966), the sequence of respiratory tract bacterial colonization preceding hospital-acquired pneumonia (1969), and the relationship between the specific type of host-immune defect and specific aetiological risks in immunocompromised patients (1977). These observations provide guiding principles for developing new management approaches now and for years to come.

With this said and done, what are the future prospects for the management of respiratory infections? Some comments, in no order of priority, follow.

Diagnosis

Advances in diagnostic techniques have progressed along two parallel, but often non-complementary, tracks. Samples obtained by device-driven invasive methods, such as CT-guided thin-needle aspirate or protected-brush bronchoscopic sampling, are all too often processed without the application of newer, molecular-based probe techniques, such as PCR and fluorescein-labelled monoclonal antibodies. The future should bring sophistication in both device and probe technology but, most importantly, a marriage of the two approaches to benefit the management of serious respiratory infections.

Fluoroquinolones

The advent of a new generation of fluoroquinolone antibiotics with enhanced (often four-fold or more) activity against *S. pneumoniae* isolates is exciting news. Quinolones have always represented an interesting class of agents for empirical treatment of community-acquired pneumonia and bronchitis; their spectrum of activity includes most of the usual respiratory pathogens, such as *Mycoplasma, Chlamydia, Legionella* and *H. influenzae* (including beta-lactamase-producing strains). The major concern with earlier agents, such as ciprofloxacin and ofloxacin has been the relatively high drug concentrations needed to suppress *S. pneumoniae* (e.g. minimum inhibitory concentrations, MICs, ≥ 1.0 mg/litre in most reports). With the newer quinolones, such as sparfloxacin, moxifloxacin, trovafloxacin, levoflaxacin, gattifloxacin and grepafloxacin, the reported MICs for *S. pneumoniae* are often less than 0.25 mg/litre. In fact, if one is a believer in the clinical (not microbiological) importance of emerging penicillin resistance among respiratory *S. pneumoniae* isolates, it is encouraging to note that *in-vitro* testing of the new fluoroquinolones against these isolates suggests that clinical activity should be acceptable. Larger clinical trials will be needed to confirm this hopeful prediction. Do these new fluoroquinolones, then, represent the 'perfect' empirical agent for community-acquired pneumonia? Or will overuse due to their enthusiastic acceptance lead to the emergence of unpleasant resistance patterns? Time will tell.

Hospital-acquired pneumonia

A major challenge for the future in dealing with the discouraging problem of hospital-acquired pneumonia is to develop data to clarify the relative benefits, risks, and cost-effective outcomes for:

- invasive diagnostic approaches, such as protected-brush bronchoscopic sampling or bronchial lavage
- prophylactic, selective antibiotic decontamination strategies, such as oral non-absorbable antibiotics and/or topically applied antibiotics.

These two management tools have been touted recently, in some cases in controlled studies, to improve diagnostic accuracy and to reduce the risk of pneumonia. However, false-positive and negative results are well described for the various invasive diagnostic methods, while the emergence of increased rates of Gram-positive respiratory infection in the face of prophylactic antibiotics has been reported. Most importantly, the clinical justification for the extra costs based on prospective trial designs needs to be, and we believe will be, studied carefully in the near future.

AIDS patients

From the beginning, the major target organ for opportunistic infections among people with AIDS has been the lung. What will be the impact of highly active antiretroviral therapy (HAART) on this complication? The good news is that a trend is already evident among recipients of HAART for reduced numbers of opportunistic infections, including those of the lung. While we predict that overall this trend will continue, we are also concerned that intolerance of HAART by some patients and/or emergence of resistance to HAART, may limit this favourable trend to subpopulations of patients. Let us hope that the majority of affected individuals continue to enjoy this pattern of reduced infections.

In summary

Future trends will confirm that respiratory infections are not immune to the delicate balance of 'progress' in modern medicine. While advances in diagnostic and therapeutic modalities will be evermore sophisticated, the broad use of more invasive and immunosuppressive strategies for all kinds of diseases will surely spawn new and, in some cases, more deadly types of respiratory infection. Let us hope that the balance can remain in our favour.

Key references

COMMUNITY-ACQUIRED PNEUMONIA

American Thoracic Society. Guidelines for the initial management of adults with community-acquired pneumonia: diagnosis, assessment of severity, and initial antimicrobial therapy. *Am Rev Respir Dis* 1993;148:1418–26.

British Thoracic Society. Guidelines for the management of community-acquired pneumonia in adults admitted to hospital. *Br J Hosp Med* 1993;49:346–50.

Bartlett JG, Breiman RF, Mandell LA, File TM Jr. Community-acquired pneumonia: guidelines for management. The Infectious Diseases Society of America. *Clin Infect Dis* 1998;26:811–38.

HOSPITAL-ACQUIRED PNEUMONIA

Centres for Disease Control. Definitions for nosocomial infections 1988. *Am Rev Respir Dis* 1988;139:1058–9.

INFECTIVE EXACERBATION OF CHRONIC OBSTRUCTIVE PULMONARY DISEASE

Celli BR. Standards for the optimal management of COPD. *Chest* 1998; 113: 283S–7S.

Wilson R. The role of infection in COPD. *Chest* 1998;113:242S–8S.

Saint S, Bent S, Vittinghoff E, Grady D. Antibiotics in chronic obstructive pulmonary disease exacerbations. A meta-analysis. *JAMA* 1995;273:957–60.

PULMONARY TUBERCULOSIS

Miller FJW. *Tuberculosis in Children.* Edinburgh: Churchill Livingstone, 1982.

BRONCHIECTASIS AND CYSTIC FIBROSIS

Cole PJ, Wilson R. Host–microbial inter-relationships in respiratory infection. *Chest* 1989;95:217S–83.

PNEUMONIA IN THE IMMUNOCOMPROMISED HOST

Fanta CH, Pennington JE. Pneumonia in the immunocompromised host. In: Pennington JE, ed. *Respiratory Infections: Diagnosis and Management.* 3rd ed. New York: Raven Press, 1994:275–95.

HIV INFECTION AND PULMONARY DISEASE

Wallace JM, Hansen NI, Lavange L *et al.* Respiratory disease trends in the Pulmonary Complications of HIV Infection Study cohort. Pulmonary Complications of HIV Infection Study Group. *Am J Resp Crit Care Med* 1997;155:72–80.

MICROBIOLOGY

Read RC, Finch RG. Bacterial infections of the respiratory tract. In: Hauster WJ, Sussman M, eds. *Topley & Wilson's Microbiology amd Microbial Infections, Ninth Edition. Volume 3. Bacterial Infections.* London: Arnold, 1998:319–46.

Index